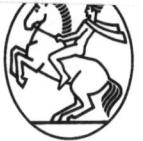

New Aspects for Treatment with Fosfomycin

Edited by
J.-P. Guggenbichler

Springer-Verlag Wien New York

Doz. Dr. Josef-Peter Guggenbichler
Universitäts-Kinderklinik Innsbruck, Austria

With 21 Figures

ISBN-13: 978-3-211-81986-9   e-ISBN-13: 978-3-7091-8903-0
DOI: 10.1007/978-3-7091-8903-0

Foreword

Fosfomycin is an antimicrobial substance which is available since several years. In earlier clinical studies an oral preparation with poor absorption in a low dosage resulted in inadequate therapeutic results. The presently used parenteral administration in a dosage range of up to 250 mg/kg BW however allowed us to appreciate several unique properties of this drug which make it valuable in the treatment of serious bacterial infections.

Due to its small molecular weight and complete lack of protein binding a favorable penetration in tissues and deep compartments (e.g., meninges, bone, heart valves) was observed. In addition fosfomycin shows a remarkably low toxicity and even protects from the nephrotoxigenic effects of aminoglycosides and other drugs. Earlier problems in antimicrobial susceptibility testing have been solved by addition of glucose 6 phosphate into the growth medium. Fosfomycin, the first representative of a completely new class of antibiotics does not show cross-resistance with other antibiotics; therefore pathogens of nosocomial infections, particularly methicillin- und gentamicin-resistant staphylococci are mostly susceptible to this antibiotic.

Clinical investigations show a favorable therapeutic outcome in severe nosocomial infections despite of previous therapeutic approaches with various other potent antibiotics.

In an international symposium in Mexico City the available clinical experience with this drug was presented and indications for the use of this antibiotic were established.

Prof. Dr. K. H. Spitzy

Contents

Summary

Presently more than 250 different antibiotics are available for clinical use and more are coming every year. Fosfomycin, the first representative of a completely new class of antibiotics with several promising theoretical advantages was introduced in Europe a few years ago. In an international symposium in Mexico City in March 1986 presently available clinical and theoretical investigations were presented and indications for fosfomycin were established. The present booklet is a summary of representative papers presented at this meeting.

The most important question arises whether there is a need and justification for a new antibiotic like fosfomycin:

From a microbiological point of view numerous antibiotics are available for the overwhelming majority of bacterial organisms. Over the last years the emergence of multiple resistant organisms and cross-resistance with many available potent new antibiotics has become a problem in the treatment of nosocomial infections. Many staphylococcal isolates in intensive care units for instance developed resistance against β lactam antibiotics including methicillin and aminoglycosides. Presently multiple resistant coagulasenegative staphylococci prevail in postoperative wound infections and these organisms are sensitive to vancomycin and/or rifampin only. Kayser presented data that fosfomycin exhibits excellent bactericidal activity against numerous multiple resistant strains of Staphylococcus aureus and its activity compares well with other available antistaphylococcal agents. Problems in antimicrobial susceptibility testing, e.g., the skip tube phenomenon should not be overemphasized as it is rare in his opinion.

From a clinical point of view there are still numerous serious life threatening bacterial infections where our therapeutic results are unsatisfactory. Several reasons account for this problem. β lactam antibiotics and aminoglycosides penetrate poorly into deep compartments, e.g., meninges, bone, myocardial tissue, heart valves, subcutaneous tissue etc. Fosfomycin with its small molecular weight and lack of protein binding shows excellent tissue penetration, which was presented in several publications (Pfeiffer, Tritthart, Achatzy).

Höger reports on the penetration of fosfomycin into macrophages and granulocytes and on the impact of fosfomycin and other antibiotics like rifampin on functional parameters, e.g., chemiluminescence, respiratory burst, phagocytosis and intracellular killing of bacteria.

These pharmacokinetic advantages and a remarkably low toxicity were the indications to try fosfomycin in the treatment of serious bacterial infections. Unlike other antibiotics which are investigated for broad clinical use, fosfomycin was intended for the treatment of difficult to treat infections, e.g., in immunocompromized patients, where presently accepted treatment regimen have failed. Indications for fosfomycin were bacterial meningitis in premature and newborn infants where a mortality of 12–25% is still seen. Fosfomycin was also used in the treatment of shunt infections where staphylococci can not be eradicated from the surface of plastic foreign bodies. The penetration of fosfomycin in meninges with little or no disturbance of the blood-brain barrier made it a valuable drug. Therapeutic studies with fosfomycin were also performed in brain abscesses, in chronic recurrent bone infections, in acute hematogenous osteomyelitis. A new pathophysiologic concept for this disorder and therapeutic implications for the use of fosfomycin and/or clindamycin was presented. Fosfomycin was also investigated in the treatment of complicated urinary tract infection, in the treatment of severe refractory pulmonary tract infections, in patients with congestive heart failure and cystic fibrosis. Virtually all patients started on fosfomycin therapy alone or in various combinations were pretreated with an accepted standard treatment without success.

It must be clear, that fosfomycin could frequently not be used as monotherapy in these seriously ill patients. Fosfomycin was combined with various β lactam antibiotics or aminoglycosides and other supportive measures. At the same time it also must be clear that a usual statistical analysis was not possible with these multifactorial, complicated case histories despite of remarkably high numbers of patients enrolled in these therapeutic trials. An alternative approach was used therefore. Most emphasis was put on the individual course of the disease after including fosfomycin in the antibiotic regimen. Under these aspects these studies seem like a number of extended pilot studies and would require confirmation by prospective, randomized, double blind trials comparing standard therapy with fosfomycin alone or in various combinations. We believe, however, that our ethical standards would not allow us to perform such studies at the present time. It is also our conviction, that therapeutic results, which are generally superior to accepted therapeutic regimen despite of a negative patient selection, allow us a fair appreciation of the therapeutic value of fosfomycin and/or the various combinations with fosfomycin, particularly in the light of previous treatment failures.

Fosfomycin exhibits a remarkably low toxicity. No hepatic, renal and hematologic side effects are described. Fosfomycin is tolerated well even when high daily doses of 5 g TID are administered. The only problem comes from its high sodium content. Electrolyte balance studies were performed.

With the exception of patients with impaired renal function, when hypokalemia was observed no other electrolyte abnormalities were noted. Determination of central venous pressure and measurements of the right ventricular diameter in patients with congestive heart failure under treatment with fosfomycin suggested a right ventricular fluid overload. Fosfomycin should be used with great care when administered to patients with right heart failure.

In conclusion it can be stated, that fosfomycin could be used in various combinations in the treatment of serious life threatening infections where previous antibiotic regimen may have failed.

Zusammenfassung

Gegenwärtig stehen uns mehr als 250 Antibiotika zur Verfügung, und jedes Jahr kommen neue hochwirksame Substanzen dazu. Fosfomycin wurde vor einigen Jahren als Breitspektrum-Antibiotikum einer völlig neuen Gruppe von antimikrobiell wirksamen Präparaten mit einer Reihe von theoretischen Besonderheiten in Europa eingeführt. Im Rahmen eines internationalen Symposiums in der Stadt Mexiko im März 1986 wurden gegenwärtig vorliegende theoretische und klinisch-therapeutische Erfahrungen mit Fosfomycin vorgestellt. Dieses Buch ist eine Zusammenfassung repräsentativer Arbeiten, die den Einsatzbereich dieses Antibiotikums festlegen.

Zuerst erhebt sich die Frage, ob eine Notwendigkeit und Berechtigung für dieses neue Antibiotikum besteht.

Wenn man das Problem von einer mikrobiologischen Sicht betrachtet, haben wir für den Großteil bakterieller Infektionen ausgezeichnet wirksame Präparate zur Verfügung. Bei im Krankenhaus erworbenen Infektionen stellt sich jedoch bereits das Problem der Resistenzentwicklung und Kreuzresistenz von Antibiotika untereinander auf zahlreiche Keime. Zum Teil stehen uns kaum noch wirksame Präparate zur Verfügung. Staphylokokken, insbesondere auf Intensivstationen, haben in den letzten Jahren zum Teil Resistenz gegen alle β-Laktam-Antibiotika (Methicillinresistenz) und Aminoglykoside entwickelt und sind nur noch auf Vancomycin und evtl. Rifampin empfindlich. Fosfomycin besitzt, wie Kayser in seiner Abhandlung zeigt, eine ausgezeichnete Wirksamkeit auf koagulasepositive und koagulasenegative Staphylokokken und besteht den Vergleich mit anderen Staphylokokkenmedikamenten gut. „Ausreißer", d. h. Keime mit natürlicher Resistenz, die die antimikrobielle Empfindlichkeitsprüfung stören, sollten wegen der Seltenheit nicht überbewertet werden.

Wenn man das Problem von einer klinischen Warte betrachtet, sind für eine Reihe schwerer, lebensbedrohlicher Infektionen, in erster Linie Infektionen in tiefen Kompartments (Meningen, Knochen), bei Infektionen immunsupprimierter Patienten und Tumorpatienten sowie bei der Mukoviszidose unbefriedigende therapeutische Ergebnisse zu verzeichnen.

Fosfomycin besitzt eine besondere Kinetik und Gewebepenetration sowie eine bemerkenswert niedrige Toxizität. Antibiotika, insbesondere β-Laktam-Antibiotika und Aminoglykoside, penetrieren vielfach schlecht in tiefe Kompartments (Meningen, Knochen) und in Granulozyten und Makrophagen. Das niedrige Molekulargewicht und die fehlende Eiweißbildung ermöglichen Fosfomycin eine überaus gute Gewebepenetration. Höger berichtet über die gute Penetration von Fosfomycin in Granulozyten und den günstigen Einfluß auf Phagozytose und intrazelluläre Abtötung von Keimen.

Fosfomycin wurde nun nicht wie die meisten anderen Neuentwicklungen auf dem Antibiotikasektor als breit wirkendes Präparat gegen diverse Infektionen eingesetzt, sondern gezielt auf Probleminfektionen, bei denen die gegenwärtig als Standard betrachtete Therapie erfolglos war, angesetzt. Bei diesen Infektionen, das sind die eitrige Meningitis bei Früh- und Neugeborenen, Shuntinfektionen, Hirnabszesse, septische, über Jahre bestehende Knocheninfektionen, schwere komplizierte Harnwegsinfektionen, pulmonale Infekte und die Mukoviszidose, jedoch auch Infektionen beim Tumorpatienten, wurde Fosfomycin in therapeutischen Untersuchungen eingesetzt.

Jedem Kliniker ist klar, daß man bei diesen lebensbedrohlich kranken Patienten, die bereits vielfach vorbehandelt waren, ein Antibiotikum nicht als Monotherapie einsetzen kann. Fosfomycin wurde deshalb meist in Kombination mit verschiedenen anderen Antibiotika (Aminoglykosiden, Cephalosporinen der 2. und 3. Generation) und zusätzlichen unterstützenden Maßnahmen (z. B. chirurgischen Eingriffen) eingesetzt. Gleichzeitig muß auch klar sein, daß eine übliche statistische Auswertung bei den vielfach kompliziert gelagerten, untereinander schwer vergleichbaren Fällen nicht möglich ist, obwohl die Fallzahlen bei den einzelnen Indikationen bemerkenswert hoch sind (100 Tumorpatienten mit Fieber, 36 Früh- und Neugeborene mit Meningitis, 31 Patienten mit

Hirnabszeß, 55 Patienten mit chronischer Osteomyelitis). Es sind also streng genommen eine Vielzahl von Pilotstudien, die in diesem Buch vorgestellt werden, und keine Untersuchung wurde nach statistischen Kriterien prospektiv, randomisiert, doppelblind vergleichend durchgeführt.

Es ist jedoch mit aller Deutlichkeit zu betonen, daß bei unseren gegenwärtigen Vorstellungen von medizinischer Ethik bei diesen schwerwiegenden Krankheitsbildern heute keine solche Vergleichsstudien mehr durchgeführt werden dürfen. Als Beurteilung mußte daher eine alternative Vorgangsweise gewählt werden: erfolglose Vorbehandlung mit einer gegenwärtig akzeptierten Standardtherapie. Bei fehlender klinischer oder bakteriologischer Besserung Umstellung auf Fosfomycin in Kombination mit verschiedenen anderen Antibiotika. Besonderes Augenmerk wurde auf den individuellen Krankheitsverlauf und die prompte klinische Besserung nach Umstellung der Antibiotikatherapie gelegt. Ein Großteil der Patienten konnte dadurch erfolgreich behandelt werden; die Ergebnisse waren insgesamt wesentlich besser, als die, die mit herkömmlichen Behandlungsschemata laut Literatur und persönlicher Erfahrung der einzelnen Autoren erwartet werden konnten. Wir glauben nun, daß uns auch diese Art der Beurteilung einen legitimen Schluß auf die Wirksamkeit des Präparates bzw. der Antibiotikakombination erlaubt.

Fosfomycin zeichnet sich durch eine besonders niedrige Toxizität aus. Einzig der hohe Natriumgehalt gibt zu Besorgnis Anlaß. In mehreren Studien, z. B. bei Patienten mit eingeschränkter Nierenfunktion, wurde die Elektrolytbilanz genau untersucht. Mit Ausnahme einer Hypokaliämie, die durch Kaliumsubstitution leicht beherrschbar war, wurden keine Elektrolytverschiebungen beobachtet. Bei Patienten mit Rechtsherzinsuffizienz wurde im zentralen Venendruck und im echokardiographisch gemessenen Rechtsherzdurchmesser Veränderungen, die auf eine akute Volumsbelastung schließen lassen, beobachtet. Bei herzdekompensierten Patienten ist daher Fosfomycin mit Vorsicht anzuwenden.

Zusammenfassend kann man festhalten, daß Fosfomycin bei

schweren, lebensbedrohlichen, bakteriellen Infektionen mit emp-
findlichen Erregern, in Kombination mit verschiedenen β-Laktam-
Antibiotika oder Aminoglykosiden therapeutische Ergebnisse er-
brachte, die mit anderen Behandlungsschemata nicht erzielbar
waren.

Activity of Fosfomycin
Against Grampositive Bacteria

H. Kayser

Institut für Medizinische Mikrobiologie der Universität Zürich, Schweiz

Summary

This review of the in vitro activity of fosfomycin against grampositive bacteria is presented in four parts:
1. An overall summary of the activity of this drug against grampositive aerobic and anaerobic organisms. The results of this investigation suggest, that the major target organism for this antimicrobial agent are staphylococci.
2. Comparison of the in vitro activity of fosfomycin with established antistaphylococcal antibiotics and other investigational drugs.
3. Demonstration of the bactericidal activity of fosfomycin against staphylococci.
4. Discussion of a unique problem, the skip tube phenomenon, observed in in vitro susceptibility testing of staphylococci to fosfomycin.

Zusammenfassung

In dieser Untersuchung werden eine Reihe verschiedener Aspekte der antimikrobiellen Empfindlichkeitsprüfung von Fosfomycin gegen grampositive Erreger beschrieben:
1. Zusammenfassung der antimikrobiellen Wirksamkeit gegen zahlreiche, größtenteils multipel resistente klinische Isolate grampositiver Kokken aus der Universitätsklinik Zürich. Untersucht wurden jeweils 100 koagulasepositive als auch koagulasenegative Stämme der Spezies Staphylokokkus, die wiederum in jeweils 50 methicillin-/gentamycinempfindliche und methicillin-/gentamycinresistente Keime aufgeschlüsselt wurden. Die Unterschiede in den MHK-Werten von Fosfomycin waren gering; der mittlere

MHK-Wert für methicillin- und gentamycinresistente koagulasepositive und koagulasenegative Staphylokokken war identisch und betrug 2.0 µg/ml. Bei den methicillin-/gentamycinempfindlichen Stämmen betrug die mittlere minimale Hemmkonzentration for koagulasepositive Stämme 1.2 µg/ml, für koagulasenegative Stämme 2.8 µg/ml, in dieser Gruppe wurden auch gelegentlich fosfomycinresistente Stämme isoliert. Die antimikrobielle Wirksamkeit von Fosfomycin gegen verschiedene Streptokokken (Lancifield A, B, C, G) und Pneumokokken war deutlich geringer und lag zwischen 20 und 97 µg/ml. Auch Enterokokken und Corynebakterien müssen als weitgehend resistent betrachtet werden. Anaerobe Streptokokken und Clostridien sind hingegen größtenteils empfindlich.

Diese Daten legen nahe, daß als Zielgruppe für Fosfomycin in erster Linie koagulasepositive und -negative Staphylokokken in Frage kommen, wobei die gute Wirksamkeit gegen resistente Keime zu betonen ist.

2. In der Folge wurde die Wirksamkeit von Fosfomycin auf Staphylokokken mit verschiedenen gebräuchlichen Staphylokokkenmedikamenten und auch mit anderen, noch in experimenteller Untersuchung stehenden Antibiotika verglichen. Fosfomycin sowie Rifampin, Fusidinsäure und Vancomycin zeigen eine Empfindlichkeit zwischen 89 und 100%. Die mittleren MHK-Werte von Rifampin (0.02 µg/ml) und Fusidinsäure (0.17 µg/ml) sind zwar im Vergleich zu Fosfomycin (1.9 µg/ml) und Vancomycin 1.1 µg/ml) niedriger, es liegen jedoch auch die Breakpoints für die beiden erstgenannten Präparate mit 2 und 4 µg/ml deutlich niedriger. Im Vergleich zu Teichoplanin, Ciprofloxacin und Coumermycin ist die Empfindlichkeit von Fosfomycin gegen diese schwer zu behandelnden Staphylokokken ebenso etwas niedriger. Auch diese neuen Antibiotika weisen wegen der geringeren Bioverfügbarkeit einen wesentlich niedrigeren Breakpoint auf.

3. Untersuchungen der Bakterizidie von Fosfomycin auf Staphylokokken zeigen eine rasche bakterizide Wirksamkeit von Fosfomycin, wobei bei Konzentrationen von 10 × MHK innerhalb von 8 Stunden eine Keimreduktion um 2 log 10 beobachtet wurde. Bei diesen Untersuchungen wurde jedoch fallweise ein Auswachsen einer kleinen Population resistenter Mikroorganismen beobachtet.

4. Die Ergebnisse der MHK-Bestimmung von Fosfomycin hängen vom Nährmedium ab. Dies hängt von der unterschiedlichen Stimulation des Hexose-6-Phosphat-Systems ab. Müller-Hinton-Bouillone soll daher durch Zugabe von 25 mg/l Glucose-6-Phosphat ergänzt werden. In der MHK-Testung in flüssigem Medium kann man das „Skip-tube-Phänomen" bisweilen beobachten, d. h. daß Bakterienwachstum in Näpfchen mit höheren Wirkstoffkonzentrationen bei Keimfreiheit in Näpfchen mit niedrigeren Konzentrationen beobachtet wird. Dieses Phänomen entsteht durch das Auswachsen fallweise resistenter Mutanten; in 2.5% aller Untersuchungen wurde dieses Phänomen beobachtet.

Zusammenfassend kann festgehalten werden, daß Fosfomycin eine ausgezeichnete Wirkung gegen verschiedene resistente Staphylokokkenstämme und eine rasche bakterizide Wirkung aufweist.

Introduction

Fosfomycin is a new antibiotic with a broad range of antimicrobial activity against grampositive and gramnegative organisms. By inhibiting one or the first steps in cell wall synthesis a rapid bactericidal activity is observed. It was of interest to investigate various aspects of in vitro susceptibility testing against grampositive organisms; many of these organisms were multiple resistant isolates from patients with hospital acquired infections. Also problems with antimicrobial susceptibility testing were further elucidated. Table 1 shows a summary of this investigation:

Table 1

---

1. Summary of the activity of fosfomycin against grampositive cocci and rods
2. Comparison of fosfomycin with other drugs against staphylococci
3. Bactericidal activity of fosfomycin against staphylococci
4. Problems with antimicrobial susceptibility testing with fosfomycin

---

Material, Methods and Results

Ad 1. Investigation of the Minimal Inhibitory Concentration

of fosfomycin against various grampositive bacteria. The mean and mode values as well as the range of MICs are presented. The MIC 50% and MIC 90% values represent the concentrations of fosfomycin inhibiting 50 and 90% of the organisms. As can be seen in Table 2, fosfomycin exhibited excellent activity against staphylococci no matter whether they are resistant to methicillin and/or gentamicin. Strains resistant to fosfomycin were rarely encountered.

The activity of fosfomycin against streptococci of groups A, B, C and G and against pneumococci was low (Table 3). Most strains

Table 2

Organism	Minimal inhibitory concentration (mg/l)				
	Mean	Mode	50%	90%	Range
Staphylococcus aureus					
Mec^S/Gen^S (N = 50)	1.2	0.5/2	1	2	0.5–32
Mec^R/Gen^R (N = 50)	2.1	2	2	4	1–8
Coagulasenegative staphylococcus					
Mec^S/Gen^S (N = 50)	2.8	1	1	1,024	0.06–1,024
Mec^R/Gen^R (N = 50)	2	2	2	4	0.25–64

Table 3

Organism	Minimal inhibitory concentration (mg/l)				
	Mean	Mode	50%	90%	Range
Streptococcus A (N = 25)	40.3	64	64	64	8–64
Streptococcus B (N = 25)	38.1	64	32	64	16–64
Streptococcus C (N = 10)	97.1	256	256	256	16–256
Streptococcus G (N = 10)	32	32	64	64	16–64
Streptococcus pneumoniae (N = 25)	20.4	32	16	64	8–128

Table 4

Organism	Minimal inhibitory concentration (mg/l)				
	Mean	Mode	50%	90%	Range
Streptococcus faecalis (N = 50)	52.3	64	64	64	32–128
Streptococcus faecium (N = 31)	70.7	64	64	128	32–512
Corynebacterium sp. (N = 60)	>256	>256	<256	<256	4–<256

Table 5

Organism	N	Number of strains with MICs (mg/l) of							
		≤0.5	1	2	4	8	16	32	≥64
Peptococcus sp.	18	—	1	8	5	1	1	1	1
Peptostreptococcus sp.	5	1	—	—	—	—	2	2	—
Cl. perfringens	4	—	—	—	—	—	—	1	3
Cl. difficile	1	—	—	—	1	—	—	1	—
Other clostridium sp.	16	—	—	—	—	—	4	4	2

Data taken from Vömel et al. (1981).

could only be inhibited by concentrations of 32 and 64 mg/l and must thus be considered as moderately resistant. MICs of more than 64 mg/l characterize a strain as resistant.

With mode MICs of 64 mg/l against Streptococcus fecalis and Streptococcus faecium this drug exhibits only very limited activity against the enterococci (Table 4). Corynebacteria isolated as possible pathogens from immunocompromised patients were resistant to fosfomycin.

The anaerobic peptococci were as susceptible to the drug as staphylococci whereas the peptostreptococci and various clostridia showed only moderate activity (Table 5).

Ad 2. Comparison of Fosfomycin with Other Drugs

From the data presented above it can be concluded that the major grampositive target group of fosfomycin is that of staphylococci. We therefore examined the activity of fosfomycin against a special collection of multiple resistant staphylococci—all of which were resistant to methicillin, many also to gentamicin—and compared the agent with other antistaphylococcal drugs (Table 6). Our data show that fosfomycin is as active as vancomycin on a weight per weight basis. Fusidic acid and rifampicillin, however, are 10–100 times more active than the former drugs. All strains were susceptible to vancomycin. The percentage of strains susceptible to the other agents varied, depending of the local application of these drugs. Ninety percent of these difficult-to-treat organisms were susceptible to fosfomycin.

We also examined the activity of some investigational drugs not yet licensed worldwide (Table 7). Activity of teicoplanin, the quinolone derivative ciprofloxacin and coumermycin was excellent and strains resistant to these antibiotics were only occasionally observed.

Ad 3. Bactericidal Activity of Fosfomycin

Fosfomycin is a drug with a good bactericidal activity against staphylococci. Timekill curves usually showed reduction of colony

Table 6. Staphylococcus aureus (N = 44); Coagulasenegative staphylococci (N = 37)

Drug	MIC (mg/l)				Susceptible breakpoint	Susceptible strains (%)
	Mean	Mode	50%	90%		
Fosfomycin	1.9	2	2	16	⩽16	90
Fusidic acid	0.17	0.12	0.12	2	⩽4	99
Rifampin	0.02	0.01	0.01	8	⩽2	89
Vancomycin	1.1	2	1	2	⩽4	100

Table 7. Staphylococcus aureus (N = 44); Coagulasenegative staphylococci (N = 37)

Drug	MIC (mg/l)				Susceptible breakpoint	Susceptible strains (%)
	Mean	Mode	50%	90%		
Teicoplanin	0.48	0.5	0.5	1	⩽4	100
Ciprofloxacin	0.25	0.25	0.25	1	⩽1	99
Coumermycin	0.01	0.02	0.01	0.03	⩽2	100

Table 8. Bactericidal activity of fosfomycin against staphylococci

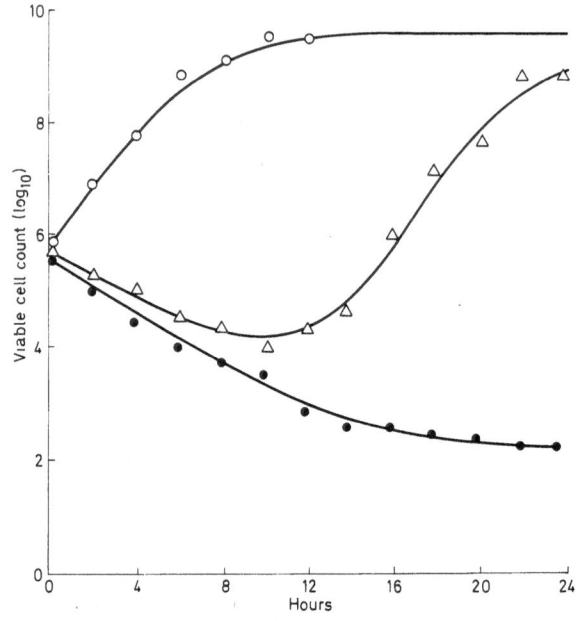

○——○ Control, ●——● 10 × MIC of fosfomycin, △——△ 10 × MIC
of fosfomycin, outgrowth of preformed mutant organisms.

forming units after 8 hours by more than 2 logs (Table 8). After
further incubation the number of viable cells was further reduced.
Occasionally regrowth occurred after 12 hours of incubation. This
phenomenon was caused by the outgrowth of a small number of
preformed resistant mutant cells in the inoculum.

Ad 4. Bacteriological Problems with Fosfomycin Susceptibility Testing

MIC test results of fosfomycin can vary with the test medium in use.
This variation is due to a different induction of the hexose-6-
phosphate transport system responsible for the permeation of
fosfomycin through the cytoplasmic membrane. Mueller-Hinton

Table 9. Bacteriological problems with fosfomycin

Variability of test results in relation to the growth medium used

Supplementation of Mueller-Hinton medium with glucose-6-phosphate (25 mg/l)

Induction of the hexose-6-phosphate transport system

Skip tube/well phenomenon in broth dilution tests

○	○	●	○	○	●	●	●	
256	128	64	32	16	8	4	2	mg/l

○	clear	tubes (cells)
●	turbid	

Table 10

Number (%) of tests without skips	Number (%) of tests with 1 skipped well	Number (%) of tests with 2 or more skipped wells
71 (= 90%)	6 (= 7.5%)	2 (= 2.5%)

Micro broth dilution test (NCCLS procedure). Staphylococcus aureus: N = 45; Coagulase negative staphylococcus: N = 34.

test media should be supplemented with 25 mg/l of glucose-6-phosphate in order to obtain reliable and reproducible results. In broth dilution tests the skip tube or well phenomenon is occasionally observed (Table 9).

This phenomenon indicates growth at higher concentrations followed by no growth in tubes or wells containing lower concentrations of the drug and is due to the occasional outgrowth of resistant mutants.

We examined a collection of staphylococci in micro broth dilution for the presence of this phenomenon. Only 2.5% of the tests showed this phenomenon with 2 or more skipped wells (Table 10). The clinical relevance of this phenomenon is not yet known.

Table 11. Summary: Fosfomycin against grampositive bacteria

Good activity against staphylococci
Moderate or no activity against streptococci and grampositive anaerobes
Bactericidal activity against staphylococci
Media effect—skip tubes/wells

Summary

Fosfomycin is a drug with good activity against staphylococci including multiple resistant strains. The drug shows moderate activity or resistance against streptococci including the enterococci and against grampositive anaerobes. Fosfomycin is bactericidal against staphylococci in time-kill curve tests. Occasionally regrowth after 12 hours of incubation is observed which is due to the outgrowth of resistant mutant cells in the inoculum. Resistant mutants also are responsible for the skip tube phenomenon which can be observed in broth dilution, but not in agar dilution tests. Addition of glucose-6-phosphate to the test medium is mandatory for susceptibility testing (Table 11).

Author's address: Prof. Dr. H. Kayser, Institut für Medizinische Mikrobiologie, Universität Zürich, Gloriastrasse 32, CH-8028 Zürich, Switzerland.

Influence of Intracellularly Active Antibiotics (Fosfomycin, Rifampin, Sulfamethoxazole, Trimethoprim) on Normal Neutrophil Function in vitro

P. H. Höger

Universitäts-Kinderklinik Zürich, Switzerland, and Universitäts-Kinderklinik Würzburg, Federal Republic of Germany

Summary

In previous studies, fosfomycin (FOS), rifampin (RIF), sulfamethoxazole (SMZ) and trimethoprim (TMP) have been shown to accumulate within polymorphonuclear leukocytes (PMN, neutrophils) and to be active against intracellular staphococci. In order to investigate wheter intracellular accumulation of these agents influences normal PMN function, several important parameters (chemiluminescence, O_2-comsumption and generation of superoxide-anion ($O_2{}^-$) by stimulated PMN, chemotaxis, phagocytosis) were tested in the presence of different antibiotic concentrations. FOS and SMZ significantly enhanced chemiluminescence (FOS: + 220.9% at 1000 mg/l, SMZ: + 1128.1% at 80 mg/l, $p < 0.0005$). The effect was dose-dependent and completely reversible upon removal of the agents. In case of fosfomycin, it was accompanied by increased O_2-consumption at high concentrations. Generation $O_2{}^-$ was unaffected.

In proportion to the extracellular drug concentration, RIF induced a significant drop both in chemiluminescence (18.3% at 50 mg/l) and $O_2{}^-$-generation (46.5% at 50 mg/l, $p < 0.0005$), which was reversible too. Chemotaxis was not influenced by neither of the agents and only RIF significantly reduced the rate of phagocytosed yeast particles (41.4% at 50 mg/l, $p < 0.0005$).

It remains to be established whether these in-vitro findings are relevant to immunocompromised patients in-vivo under certain conditions.

20   P. H. Höger:

Zusammenfassung

Die intrazelluläre Anreicherung von Antibiotika in Granulozyten und Makrophagen scheint bei einer Reihe von Erkrankungen mit chronischen intrazellulären Infekten eine wesentliche therapeutische Rolle zu spielen. In früheren Untersuchungen wurde die Penetration von Fosfomycin, Rifampin, Sulfamethoxazol und Trimethoprim und die intrazelluläre Anreicherung dieser Substanzen in Granulozyten beobachtet. Es besteht ein umgekehrt proportionales Verhältnis zwischen der Polarität von Antibiotika und ihrer intrazellulären Anreicherung. Lipophile Substanzen, wie Rifampin, Erythromycin, Clindamycin, Sulfamethoxazol und Trimethoprim, werden in Granulozyten angereichert, während hydrophile (polare) Präparate, wie β-Lactam-Antibiotika (Penicillin, Cephalosporine) und Aminoglykoside, nicht in Granulozyten penetrieren. Fosfomycin bildet insofern eine Ausnahme als es als hydrophile Substanz um den Faktor 1.8— 2.1 im Vergleich zu Serum in Granulozyten angereichert wird.

Untersuchungen von Granulozyten von Patienten mit chronischer Granulomatose zeigten, daß die antimikrobielle Wirksamkeit von Antibiotika erhalten bleibt. Gleichzeitig konnte man jedoch in neueren Untersuchungen beobachten, daß verschiedene Antibiotika intrazellulär einen unerwünschten Einfluß auf spezifische und unspezifische Abwehrfunktionen ausüben.

Es war nun von Interesse, den Einfluß von Fosfomycin, Rifampin, Sulfamethoxazol und Trimethoprim in unterschiedlichen Konzentrationen auf verschiedene funktionelle Parameter normaler menschlicher Granulozyten zu untersuchen.

Untersucht wurden die Chemilumineszenz und die intrazelluläre Bildung freier Sauerstoffradikale. Fosfomycin und Sulfamethoxazol steigerten die Chemilumineszenz um 220 bzw. 1128%. Die Wirkung dieser beiden Substanzen war dosisabhängig und nach Auswaschung des Präparates vollständig reversibel. Die Steigerung der Chemilumineszenz beruht wahrscheinlich auf einem extrazellulären Mechanismus. Die Bildung freier Sauerstoffradikale war durch keines dieser Präparate beeinflußt.

Im Gegensatz dazu führte Rifampin zu einer substantiellen Verringerung der Chemilumineszenz (18%) und O_2^--Generation (46.5%).

Auch der Sauerstoffverbrauch durch PMA- oder OPZ-stimulierte Granulozyten wurde untersucht; es konnte durch keines dieser Medikamente ein negativer Einfluß auf den Sauerstoffverbrauch beobachtet werden. Fosfomycin steigerte jedoch parallel zur Steigerung der Chemilumineszenz auch den Sauerstoffverbrauch in den Granulozyten.

Fosfomycin, Sulfamethoxazol und Trimethoprim zeigen keinen Einfluß auf die Chemotaxis und Phagozytose von Keimen; unter Rifampin wurde eine signifikant verminderte Phagozytose von Hefepartikeln beobachtet (41.4%).

Mit Ausnahme von Rifampin zeigte keines der untersuchten Präparate (Fosfomycin, Sulfamethoxazol und Trimethoprim) einen hemmenden Einfluß auf die Funktionen von Granulozyten. Die klinische Relevanz dieser In-vitro-Untersuchungen bei immunsupprimierten Patienten ist jedoch noch nicht bewiesen und bedarf weiterer klinischer Untersuchungen.

Introduction

Previous studies have demonstrated intracellular accumulation of antibiotics within normal human polymorphonuclear leucocytes (PMN, neutrophils) as being indirectly proportional to the polarity of the agents [6, 7, 16]. Lipophilic antibiotics such as rifampin (RIF), erythromycin, clindamycin, sulfamethoxazole (SMZ) and trimethoprim (TMP) are concentrated passively within the cells whereas hydrophilic (polar) agents such as β lactam antibiotics (penicillin, cephalosporines) and aminoglycosides are not. Fosfomycin (FOS) although structurally hydrophilic accumulates well within PMN, probably due to active transport mechanisms [6, 10].

PMN from patients with chronic granulomatous disease (CGD) are unable to kill phagocytosed catalse-positive bacteria (e.g. staphylococci) and studies have shown that intracellularly accumulated antibiotics retain their bactericidal activity within these cells compensating for their bactericidal defect [6, 7].

While intracellular accumulation of antibiotics is a desirable property in the case of chronic intracellular infections, inhibition of normal PMN function by these agents could be detrimental especially to patients with impaired immunity (immunodeficiency disorders, granulocytopenia, cancer patients under treatment).

In this study we investigated the influence of different concentrations of FOS, RIF, SMZ and TMP at different concentrations on normal human PMN in vitro. Spontaneous and directed migration (chemotaxis), phagocytosis of yeast particles and parameters associated with the most crucial event in killing phagocytosed pathogens—the "respiratory burst"—were separately analysed.

Material and Methods

Preparation of PMN

Venous blood (20–100 ml) was drawn from healthy volunteers. PMN were isolated across a density gradient as described in the literature, resuspended in Hank's balanced salt solution (HBSS) and adjusted to the specific cell concentration required [6, 7].

Effects of Antibiotics on Normal PMN Function

Functional assays were performed in the presence of FOS[1] (25, 50, 100, 200, 400, 1,000 mg/l), RIF[2] (5, 10, 20, 50 mg/l), SMZ[3] (20, 80 mg/l) and TMP[3] (1, 5 mg/l). Concentrations were choosen according to therapeutic plasma concentrations with one concentration 2–3 times higher than maximal plasma levels. Penicillin[4] (100 and 400 mg/dl) was tested for comparison in some assays. Results with and without antibiotics were compared.

Measurement of Chemiluminescence (CL)

During the "respiratory burst" stimulated PMN release chemically reactive oxygen derivatives such as O_2^-, H_2O_2, $^1O_2$, OH^- etc. They oxydize luminol (5-amino-2,3-di-hydro-1,4-phthalazinedione, final concentration: 5×10^{-4} M, Sigma, St. Louis/Mo., USA), a cyclic hydrazide, to the electronically excited aminophthalate ion which emits photons recorded as CL when relaxing to the ground state [1, 2]. PMN (1×10^7) were activated with either a soluble (phorbol-myristate-acetate, PMA) or a particulate stimulus (opsonized zymosan, OPZ, both fromSigma). Tests were performed in a liquid scintillation photometer (Luminometer 1251, LKB Wallac, Turku, Finland) and recorded graphically. Results were expressed in mV/min/10^6 PMN.

In some experiments either sn-glycero-3-phosphate (sn-g-3-P,

---

[1] Boehringer Mannheim, Mannheim, FRG.
[2] Sodium salt, Ciba Geigy, Basle, Switzerland.
[3] Wellcome, Basle, Switzerland.
[4] Penicillin sodium, Sigma Pharm.

1 mM) or D-glucose-6-phosphate (D-g-6-P, 0.1 mM) were added to study their influence on CL in the presence of fosfomycin. In order to investigate the reversibility of the antibiotic's influence on CL the agents were removed from the PMN by washing the cells three times in HBSS 10 minutes after exposure. CL was subsequently recorded.

Production of Superoxide-Anion (O_2^-)

PMN (3×10^7/ml) were stimulated by either PMA or OPZ. Release of O_2^- was assayed by measuring the reduction of ferricytochrome c in a UV spectrophotometer (CARY 251, Varian Inc., Victoria, Australia) [4]. Results were expressed in nmol O_2^-/min/10^6 PMN. Influence of sn-g-3-P and D-g-6-P in the presence of FOS and reversibility of effects were investigated as described above.

Consumption of Oxygen (O_2)

O_2 consumption by PMA- or OPZ-stimulated PMN (5×10^6/ml) was investigated using a Clark electrode and recorded with an oxygraph (no. 5/6 H, Gilson Medical Electronics, Middleton, Ill., USA). Results were measured in nmol O_2/min/5×10^6 PMN (13).

Chemotaxis

Spontaneous migration and directed migration (chemotaxis) towards zymosan-activated serum (Sigma) of PMN (1×10^8/ml) under agarose was tested as described above [11].
   Results were expressed in μm (2 h/37°C/5% CO_2).

Phagocytosis

Phagocytosis of yeast cells (Saccharomyces cerevisae, 2.5×10^8/ml, Sigma) by PMN (5×10^6/ml) was tested as described before [7]. The mean number of phagocytosed yeast cells per 100 PMN (30 min/37 °C) was determined.

Statistical Analysis

Statistical probability was tested with Student's t test.

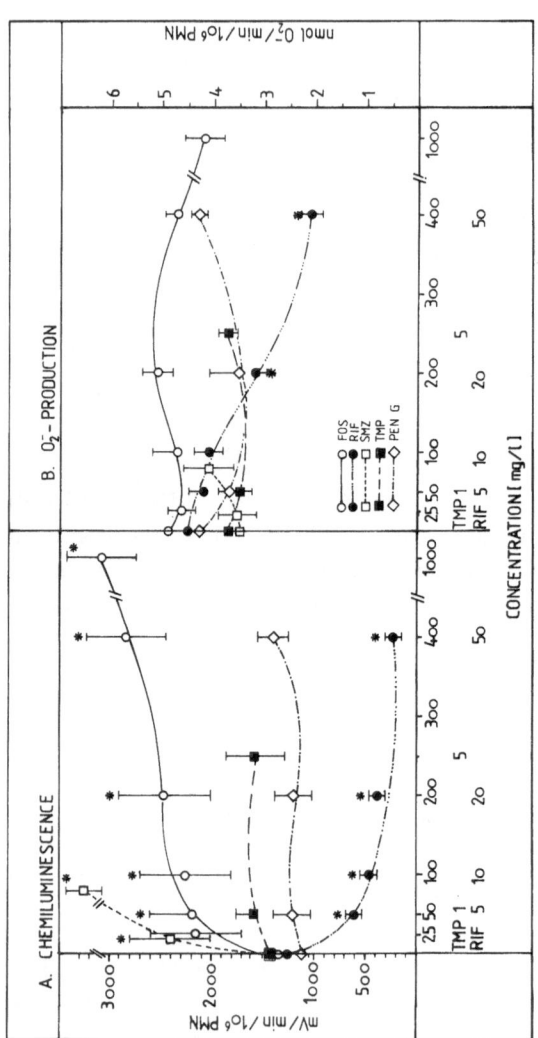

Fig. 1. Influence of antibiotics on CL and O_2^- production of stimulated normal human PMN. A Chemiluminescence: Means ± SEM, *FOS* 12–21 single determinations per concentration, *SMZ* 8–11 determinations, *TMP* 8–11 determinations, *RIF* 18 determinations, *PEN* 3–5 determinations. **B** O_2^- production: Means ± SEM, *FOS* 7–8, *TMP* 7, *SMZ* 6, *RIF* 7–12, *PEN* 3–4 single determinations per concentration. Stimulus: PMA

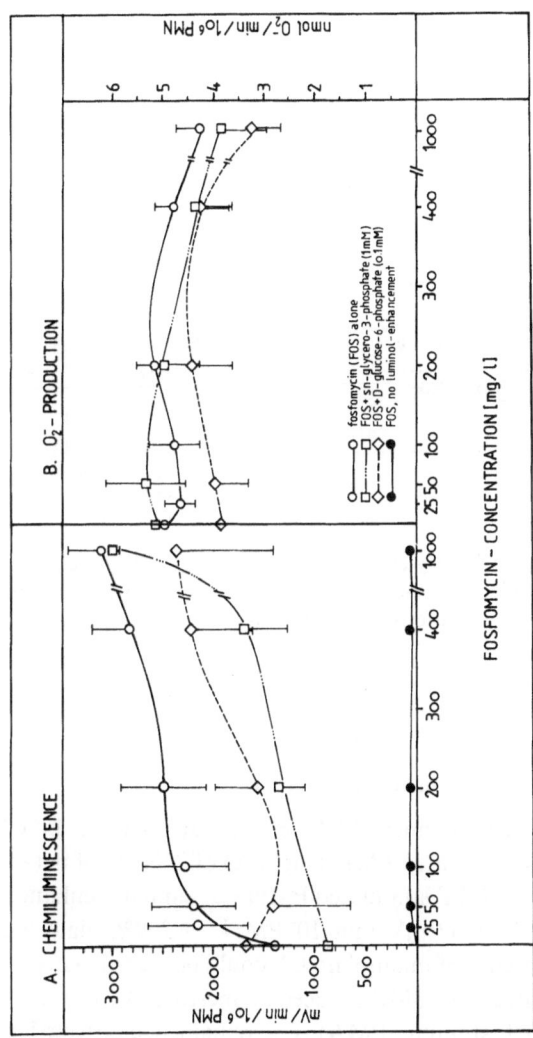

Fig. 2. Influence of fosfomycin on CL and O_2^{--} production of stimulated PMN: Effect of sn-glycero-3-P and D-glucose-6-P. Normal human PMN. Stimulus: PMA. **A** Chemiluminescence: Means ± SEM, $FOS + sn\text{-}glycero\text{-}3\text{-}P$ 2–7 single determinations per concentration, $FOS + D\text{-}glucose\text{-}6\text{-}P$ 3–6 single determinations per concentration **B** O_2^{--} production: Means ± SEM, $FOS + sn\text{-}g\text{-}3\text{-}P = 3$–6 single determinations per concentration $FOS + D\text{-}g\text{-}6\text{-}P = -5$ single determinations per concentration

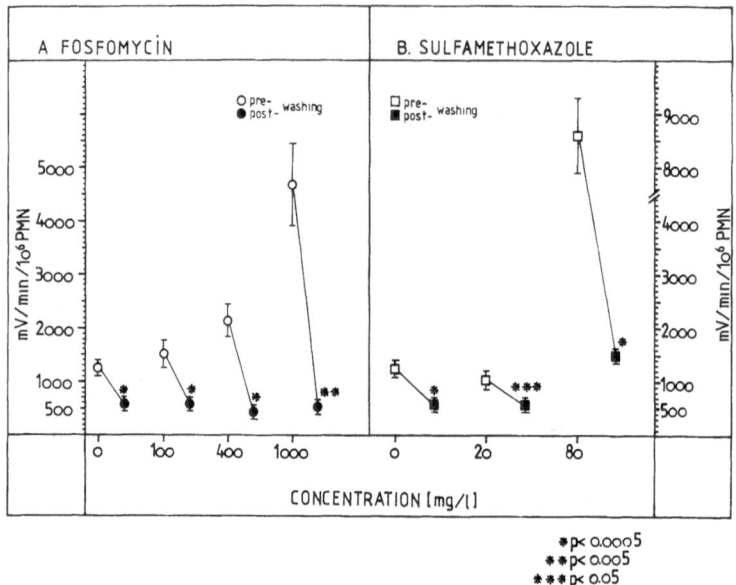

**p< 0.0005
**p< 0.005
***p< 0.05

Fig. 3. Reversal of stimulatory effect of fosfomycin and SMZ on CL. *FOS* 10–20 single determinations per concentration, *SMZ* 3–5 single determinations per concentration

Results

Chemiluminescence

In a dose-dependent manner, FOS lead to an increase in CL response of PMA stimulated PMN (Fig. 1 A) of 220.9% of net CL without FOS. CL of OPZ stimulated PMN was similarly enhanced (from 5,005 to 10,466.6 mV/min/10^6 PMN, + 209% data not shown). In the absence of luminol no CL could be recorded even at high FOS concentrations. SMZ induced an increase in CL of up to 1,128.1% (80 mg/l, stimulus PMA). CL remained unaffected by TMP and penicillin whereas RIF significantly inhibited CL in direct proportion to its extracellular concentration (Fig. 1 A); at 50 mg/l CL activity was 19.3% with PMA stimulation and 25.8% with OPZ

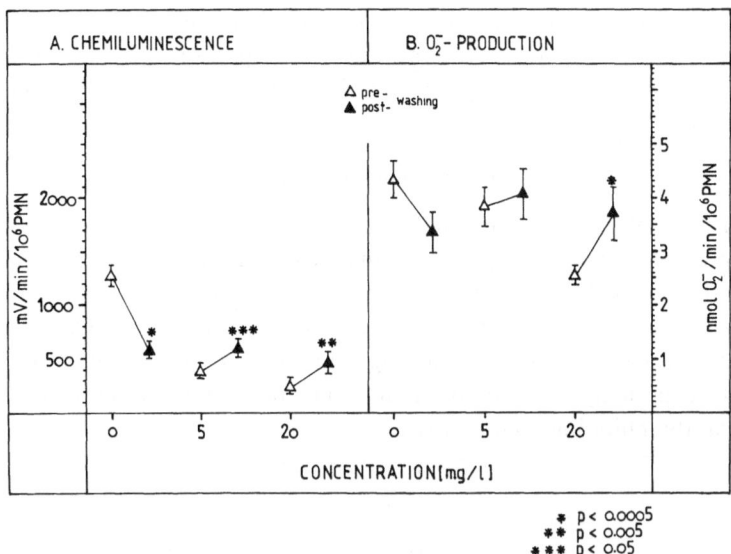

Fig. 4. Reversal of inhibitory effect of rifampin on CL and O_2^- production. CL 12–20 single determinations per concentration, O_2 8–11 single determinations per concentration

stimulation (2,414.3 mV versus 9,342.9 mV at 0 mg/l data not shown).

Both stimulatory and inhibitory effects were completely reversible (SMZ at 80 mg/l: nearly reversible) upon removal of the agents (Fig. 3 a, 3 B, 4 A).

Sn-3-g-P has been shown to inhibit intracellular accumulation of FOS probably due to competition for the same transmembranous transport channel [6, 10]. Neither this nor D-g-6-P, an inducer of another FOS transport system in bacterial cells (UDPG system), showed any significant influence on the enhancement of CL induced by FOS (Fig. 2 A).

O_2-Generation

In contrast to CL none of the agents under investigation influenced the amount of O_2-released by stimulated PMN (Fig. 1 B). One exception was RIF whose dose dependent diminution of O_2-release[5] was completely reversible (as was CL response) (Fig. 1 B, 4 B). Again sn-g-3-P and D-g-6-P did not influence the effect of FOS on PMN.

Further PMN Functional Parameters

Effects of the antibiotics on O_2 consumption, chemotaxis and yeast phagocytosis of PMN are summarized in Table 1. No negative effects on O_2 consumption and chemotaxis were observed. Increased CL in the presence of high concentrations of FOS was paralleled by a significant augmentation of O_2 consumption. Unexpectedly RIF did not diminish O_2 consumption while significantly inhibiting phagocytosis.

Discussion

Previous reports have shown that antimicrobial agents can cause various side effects on cells of the bodys own defense system [16]. Clinical practice however shows, that the use of antibiotics in the past has not resulted in an increase in severe infections due to impairment of host defense. Under normal circumstances, minor inhibition of lymphocyte or PMN function remains undetected. However, antibiotic modulation of PMN function could be of importance for patients with congenital or acquired impairment of neutrophil function or neutropenia. This group is already predisposed to infections and frequently receives long time (and high dose) antibiotic regimens. In the studies recorded here, FOS and SMZ reversibly enhanced CL of stimulated normal human PMN (Fig. 1 A). At high concentrations FOS induced a parallel increase in O_2 consumption (Table 1).

Previously an SMZ analog was shown to have an immunostimulatory effect by eliminating intracellular bacteria in CGD PMNs (9).

---

[5] At 50 mg/l: 46.5% of the baseline value in case of PMA stimulation; 36.3% = 0.368 nmol O_2^-/min/10^6 PMN in case of OPZ stimulation.

Table 1. Influence of intracellularly accumulating antibiotics on yeast-phagocytosis, chemotaxis and oxygen-consumption by stimulated normal human PMN

Antibiotic	Concentration (mg/l)	Phagocytosis (phagocytosed yeast particles/100 PMN)	Chemotaxis		O_2 consumption (nmol O_2/h/5 × 10⁶ PMN)
			Activated (μm)	Spontaneous (μm)	
FOS	0	990 ± 33.1 (6)	428 ± 47	179 ± 29 (24)	1,458.4 ± 124.5 (11)
	50	936.7 ± 31.9 (6)	338 ± 38	148 ± 20 (14)	1,214.4 ± 118.4 (8)
	100	971.7 ± 39.9 (6)	358 ± 38	156 ± 28 (15)	1,453.6 ± 207.9 (8)
	200	990.3 ± 24 (6)	387 ± 44	156 ± 19 (14)	1,356.9 ± 118 (8)
	400	945 ± 29.2 (6)	410 ± 35	141 ± 22 (16)	1,389 ± 113.3 (8)
	1,000	958.8 ± 18.6 (5)	379 ± 54	140 ± 19 (14)	1,827** ± 90.3 (8)
RIF	0	798.7 ± 20.3 (14)	663 ± 45	290 ± 26 (13)	1,662.9 ± 194.2 (7)
	5	593.7* ± 46.3 (14)	785 ± 46	302 ± 29 (10)	1,898 ± 174.5 (6)
	10	446.3* ± 82 (8)	634 ± 50	309 ± 33 (9)	1,856.6 ± 158.7 (7)
	20	541.9* ± 65.1 (14)	697 ± 56	278 ± 30 (13)	1,707.4 ± 118.3 (7)
	50	330.7* ± 57.6 (7)	573 ± 32	412 ± 21 (6)	1,827.4 ± 279.5 (7)
SMZ	0	798.7* ± 20.3 (14)	663 ± 45	290 ± 26 (13)	1,167.4 ± 175.6 (5)
	20	802 ± 23 (5)	810 ± 99	218 ± 22 (4)	1,155.4 ± 144.3 (5)
	80	882.1 ± 53.7 (7)	747 ± 69	218 ± 21 (4)	982.6 ± 97.2 (5)
TMP	0	798.7 ± 20.3 (14)	663 ± 45	290 ± 26 (13)	1,167.4 ± 175.63 (5)
	1	787 ± 32 (5)	705 ± 83	171 ± 22 (6)	1,142.2 ± 178.9 (5)
	5	783.8 ± 22.6 (8)	694 ± 114	193 ± 18 (6)	1,084.4 ± 161.3 (5)

Numbers in brackets refer to number of experiments.
* $p < 0.0005$.
** $p < 0.025$.

The exact mechanism of this immunostimulation remained undefined. Later studies revealed an inhibition of postphagocytic iodination by SMZ and TMP [3]. High concentrations (> 100 mg/l) of the agents were used in these studies and the effects were not reproducible in vivo. Inhibition of CL by SMZ and TMP was reported by others [14]. The concentration of luminol is directly proportional to the intensity of CL [5]. Significant lower luminol concentrations were used in the study mentioned and could account for the discrepancy of our findings. Using a concentration similar to ours Oleske et al. also observed a significant SMZ induced increase of CL [12].

Oxidation of microbial cell walls by O_2-radicals is followed by emission of light during relaxation to the ground state. Enhancement of CL cannot simply be explained by increased generation of O_2^- (Fig. 1 B). Other O_2 derivatives could account for it ($^1O_2$, OH^-) but the most likely explanation for this phenomenon is a luminol-like activity inherent to both FOS and SMZ. Without luminol as cofactor there is no measurable CL response. The phenomenon of CL enhancement can even be observed in the presence of sn-g-3-P and D-g-6-P which interfer with intracellular uptake of FOS [6]. Thus CL stimulation is probably caused by an extracellular mechanism.

The search for immunostimulatory agents has revealed a number of substances able to enhance oxidative metabolism. For instance Ismail et al. reported improvement of in vitro bacterial killing by a dapsone derivative. These as well as experiments with glucose oxidase coupled latex particles (increased intracellular production of H_2O_2) and with methylene blue (stimulates hexose-monophosphate-shunt) either failed to improve bactericidal activity of CGD-PMN or even proved detrimental to healthy tissue.

Continuous prophylactic therapy with SMZ/TMP in CGD patients considerably reduced the rate and severity of infections (15). It remains to be seen whether this effect can be attributed to enhanced PMN CL and whether it can be achieved by FOS as well.

Conversely the inhibitory effect of RIF on CL response and O_2^- production of activated PMN could be detrimental to patients with impaired release of O_2^- (Fig. 1 A, B). Since it was not paralleled by a decreased consumption of O_2 (Table 1) and could be demonstrated in a cell-free system as well, this inhibition can most probably be attributed to an ion-scavenging effect and not to an inhibition of the O_2^- producing enzymes.

Both stimulation of CL by FOS and SMZ and inhibition by RIF were reversible. Full restoration of normal PMN function was obtained after removal of the agents (Figs. 3 and 4). Only functional interference without cellular damage seems to occur.

Only RIF exerted a negative influence on yeast phagocytosis. Further studies are necessary to analyze whether this is due to interaction with complement receptors on the PMN surface or to other mechanisms.

None of the substances had any impact on PMN migration in vitro (Table 1).

Except for RIF intracellularly accumulated antibiotics (FOS, SMZ, TMP) revealed no inhibitory effect on normal PMN function. The inhibitory effect of RIF on CL and O_2^- release and the stimulatory effect of SMZ and FOS on CL alone are not necessarily associated with their intracellular accumulation. The in vivo significance of these findings for immunocompromised patients remains to be established. In order to avoid falsely positive (elevated) results in diagnostic CL assays, patients should discontinue FOS and SMZ 1–2 days before the test.

References

1. Allen RC, Stjernholm RL, Steele RH (1972) Evidence for the generation of electronic excitation state(s) in human polymorphonuclear leukocytes and its participation in bactericidal activity. Biochem Biophys Res Comm 47: 679–684
2. Allen RC, Loose LD (1976) Phagocytic activation of a luminol-dependent chemiluminescence in rabbit alveolar and peritoneal macrophages. Biochem Biophys Res Comm 69: 245–252
3. Anderson R, Grabow G, Oosthuizen T, Theron A, van Rensburg AJ (1980) Effects of sulfamethoxazole and trimethoprim on human

neutrophil and lymphocyte functions in vitro: in vivo effects of co-trimoxazole. Antimicrob Agents Chemother 17: 322–326

4. Babior BM, Kipnes RS, Curnutte JT (1973) The production by leukocytes of superoxide, a potential bactericidal agent. J Clin Invest 52: 741–744

5. Briheim GS, Stendahl O, Dahlgren C (1984) Intra- and extracellular events in luminol-dependent chemiluminescence of polymorpho-nuclear leukocytes. Infect Immun 45: 1–5

6. Höger PH, Seger RA, Schaad UB, Hitzig WH (1985) Chronic granulomatous disease: Uptake and intracellular activity of fosfomycin in granulocytes. Pediatr Res 19: 38–44

7. Höger PH, Vosbeck K, Seger R, Hitzig WH (1985) Uptake, intra-cellular activity, and influence of rifampin on normal function of polymorphonuclear leukocytes. Antimicrob Agents Chemother 28: 667–674

8. Ismail G, Boxer LA, Allen JM, Baehner RL (1978) Improvement of polymorphonuclear leukocyte oxidative and bactericidal functions in chronic granulomatous disease with 4-amino-4-hydroxylamino-diphenyl sulphone. Br J Haematol 40: 219–229

9. Johnston RB, Wilfert CM, Buckley RH, Webb LS, DeChatelet LR, McCall CE (1975) Enhanced bactericidal activity of phagocytes from patients with chronic granulomatous disease in the presence of sulphisoxazole. Lancet i: 824–827

10. Kahan FM, Kahan JS, Cassidy PJ, Kropp H (1974) The mechanism of action of fosfomycin (phosphonomycin). Ann NY Acad Sci 235: 364–386

11. Nelson RD, Quie PG, Simmons RL (1975) Chemotaxis under agarose: A new and simple method for measuring chemotaxis and spontaneous migration of human polymorphonuclear leukocytes and monocytes. J Immunol 115: 1650–1656

12. Oleske JM, de la Cruz A, Ahdiek H, Sorrino D, LaBraico J, Cooper R, Singh R, Lin R, Minnefor A (1983) Effects of antibiotics on polymor-phonuclear leukocyte chemiluminescence and chemotaxis. J Antimi-crob Chemother 12 [Suppl] C: 35–38

13. Segal AW, Coade B (1978) Kinetics of oxygen-consumption by phagocytizing human neutrophils. Biochem Biophys Res Commun 84: 611–617

14. Siegel JP, Remington JS (1982) Effect of antimicrobial agents on chemiluminescence of human polymorphonuclear leukocytes in re-sponse to phagocytosis. J Antimicrob Chemother 10: 505–515

15. Weening RS, Kabel P, Pijman P, Roos D (1983) Continuous therapy with sulfamethoxazole-trimethoprim in patients with chronic granu-lomatous disease. J Pediatr 103: 127–130

16. Yourtee EL, Root RK (1982) Antibiotic-neutrophil interactions in microbial killing. In: Gallin JL, Fauci AS (eds) Advances in host defense mechanisms, vol I. Raven Press, New York, pp 187–209

Author's address: Dr. P. H. Höger, Neugeborenenstation, Universitäts-Kinderklinik Hamburg, Martinistrasse 52, D-2000 Hamburg, Federal Republic of Germany.

Investigation of Fosfomycin Concentrations in the Cerebrospinal Fluid (CSF) and Its Clinical Significance in Neurosurgical Patients

G. Pfeifer, C. Frenkel, U. Hörnchen und *F. Bartels*

Universitätsklinik für Anästhesiologie (Director: Prof. Dr. H. Stöckel),
Bonn, Federal Republic of Germany

Summary

Fosfomycin is a promising antimicrobial agent for prophylaxis and therapy of central nervous system infections in neurosurgical and polytraumatized patients. It suggests itself as clinically significant since it effects a broad spectrum of microorganisms, has a low toxicity and a favorable physicochemical state (molecular weight 182, complete lack of protein binding). Although there are preliminary informations on CSF penetration of fosfomycin into the CSF a thorough analysis seemed warranted.

The investigation was carried out in 45 neurosurgical patients in whom an intraoperative or therapeutic postoperative CSF drainage was required. The blood brain barrier with normal total CSF protein and cell count in these patients was largely intact. 5 or 10 g fosfomycin was administered in 30 minute infusions. 3–6 hours after infusion with 5 g fosfomycin the CSF concentration formed a plateau between 8.6 and 11.6 µg/ml. By increasing the dose to 10 g fosfomycin the time period in which a sufficient CSF concentration was established could be markedly shortened reaching a plateau between 1 and 6 hours after infusion with peaks of 15.5 and 17.7 µg/ml. 3×5 g fosfomycin/day maintained therapeutic fosfomycin concentrations in CSF. The CSF/serum ratio determined by the area under the concentration curve was 9% after administration of 5 g and 14% after administration of 10 g fosfomycin.

4 patients with meningeal inflammation and consequent blood-brain

barrier disturbances exhibited fosfomycin concentrations 100 to 250% higher than in the healthy control group. In our analysis fosfomycin was able to penetrate the intact blood brain barrier system satisfactorily. The penetration across inflamed meninges is greatly enhanced.

Zusammenfassung

Fosfomycin eignet sich aufgrund mehrerer Besonderheiten — dem breiten antimikrobiellen Wirkungsspektum, der niedrigen Toxizität und der guten Liquorpenetration auch bei intakter Blut-Liquor-Schranke — in der Prophylaxe und Therapie von Infektionen des Zentralnervensystems beim polytraumatisierten und postoperativen Patienten. Die gute Liquorpenetration beruht vor allem auf dem kleinen Molekulargewicht dieser Substanz und der fehlenden Einweißbildung.

Obwohl bereits einzelne vorläufige Daten, die eine günstige Liquorpenetration von Fosfomycin erwarten lassen, vorliegen, wurde in dieser Untersuchung die Liquorkinetik von Fosfomycin bei 45 neurochirurgischen Patienten mit externer Ableitung intraoperativ bzw. postoperativ nochmals eingehend untersucht. Beim Großteil der Patienten bestand keine entzündliche Veränderung der Blut-Liquor-Schranke, in weiteren Untersuchungen wurde Fosfomycin therapeutisch eingesetzt.

5 und 10 g Fosfomycin wurden bei den einzelnen Patienten als Kurzinfusion über 30 Minuten verabreicht und aus der externen Abteilung des Ventrikelliquors die Konzentrationen von Fosfomycin mittels eines biologischen Testsystems bestimmt.

Nach Gabe von 5 g Fosfomycin wurde nach 3—5 Stunden ein Plateau zwischen 8.6 und 11.6 µg/ml Liquor beobachtet. Bei Gabe von 10 g Fosfomycin wurde das Plateau bereits nach 1 Stunde erreicht und lag ca. 5 Stunden lang zwischen 15,5 und 17,7 µg/ml. Die Gabe von 3×5 g Fosfomycin führte zu einem Steady state mit therapeutisch wirksamen Liquorkonzentrationen. Das Verhältnis der Liquorkonzentration zur Serumkonzentration, gemessen an der Fläche unter der Konzentrationskurve, betrug 9% (Gabe von 5 g Fosfomycin) und 14% (Gabe von 10 g Fosfomycin) bei nicht enzündlich veränderten Meningen.

Bei 4 Patienten mit eitriger Meningitis wurden ebenso Liquorkonzentrationen von Fosfomycin bestimmt. Die Penetration von Fosfomycin in entzündlich veränderte Meningen war um 100 bis 250% höher.

Zusammenfassend kann man festhalten, daß Fosfomycin ausreichend in nicht entzündlich veränderte Meningen penetriert und zu prophylaktisch bzw. therapeutisch wirksamen Liquorkonzentrationen führt. Bei entzündlich veränderten Meningen werden therapeutische Liquorkonzentrationen erzielt.

Introduction

For therapy of infections in neurosurgical patients there is a need for antibiotics characterized by good CSF penetration, high efficacy on multiresistant nosocomial microorganisms and low toxicity. Infections of the central nervous system are always acutely life threatening.

Good penetration of an antibiotic through the blood-brain barrier or blood cerebrospinal fluid (CSF) barrier is necessary to establish an adequate antibiotic concentration as quickly as possible. In order to maintain its high concentration when inflammation and permeability of the blood-brain barrier begins to recede an antibiotic must be capable to penetrate an intact barrier, a characteristic also necessary for prophylactic use.

The penetration into the CSF depends on various factors. There are substance specific factors like the degree of lipid solubility, ionization, protein binding, molecular size and steric configuration. The low relative molecular mass (molecular weight 182) and lack of protein binding enable good penetration of fosfomycin into the CSF.

Posttraumatic and postoperative meningitis is often caused by nosocomial multiresistant pathogens in contrast to the infectious meningitis, where usually readily controllable microorganisms are found.

During 1982 and 1983 we mainly identified coagulase negative staphylococci, S. aureus and Pseudomonas aeruginosa in the CSF of 72 neurosurgical patients. Fosfomycin can be classified as broad spectrum antibiotic covering many important grampositive and gramnegative organisms.

Since more than 30% of neurosurgical patients are polytraumatized with multiorgan dysfunction, the need for antibiotics with a low toxicity profile is of great importance. In addition to this the polytraumatized or postoperative patient is in permanent danger of hypovolemic, hypoxic or septic shoc. Toxicity of fosfomycin on specific organ systems has not been demonstrated.

Methods

Investigations of CSF penetration were made in patients in need of intraoperative (tumor excision) or therapeutic (hydrocephalus occlusus) CSF drainage. The blood brain barrier could be regarded as essentially intact, as total CSF protein and cell count were within the normal range. 283 serum samples and 240 CSF samples from 45 patients were analyzed. The age of our patients was in a range of 18–69 years (mean 46.6 years).

The patients were divided into two groups and were given either 5 g or 10 g fosfomycin in a 30 minutes infusion. Samples were obtained according to a predetermined schedule. Concentrations of fosfomycin in serum and CSF were determined by an agar diffusion test using a plate well method. The method was sensitive down to a concentration of 0.1 µg/ml. The pharmakokinetic parameters were calculated, evaluation was made on the basis of the least-square-fitting method by an analog computer.

Results

After intravenous administration of 5 g fosfomycin in 30 minutes the following serum kinetics were found: the maximum concentration was 260 µg/ml (s = 106 µg/ml), measured 15 minutes after completion of the infusion. The computer fitted mean curve shows a concentration near the end of infusion of 340 µg/ml. Thereafter serum concentrations felt continuously similar as observed by other investigators [3] We determined a mean distribution volume of 18.5 l, a total clearance of 120 ml/min and a serum halflife of approximately 2 hours. The area under the serum concentration curve (AUC) was 420 µg/ml · h.

Measurable concentrations were found in the CSF after the end of the 30 min infusion with 5 g fosfomycin. The mean curve shows a slow rise in concentrations for the first 3 hours and a plateau phase with stable CSF concentrations lasting as long as 6 hours followed by slow elimination over several hours (Fig. 1).

The highest mean value of 10.1 µg/ml (range 8.6 to 11.6 µg/ml) was found in the period between 180 and 360 minutes. The AUC for

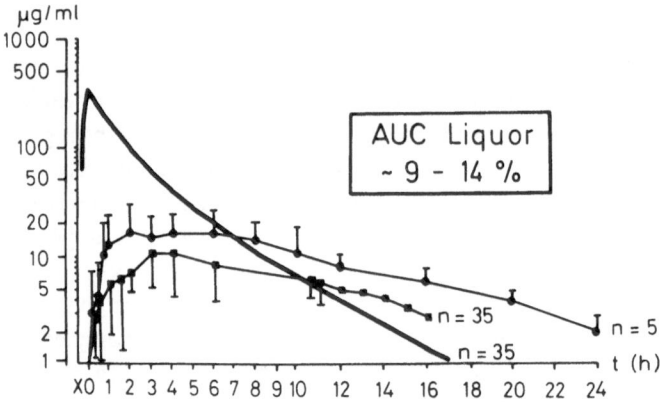

Fig. 1. Fosfomycin CSF penetration rate after a single dose in the presence of an intact blood-brain barrier (computer fitted serum curve, × begin of the infusion, 0 end of the infusion (mean values and standard deviation), —— serum concentrations after 5 g/30 min inf., ●—● liquor concentrations after 10 g/30 min inf., ■—■ liquor concentrations after 5 g/30 min inf.

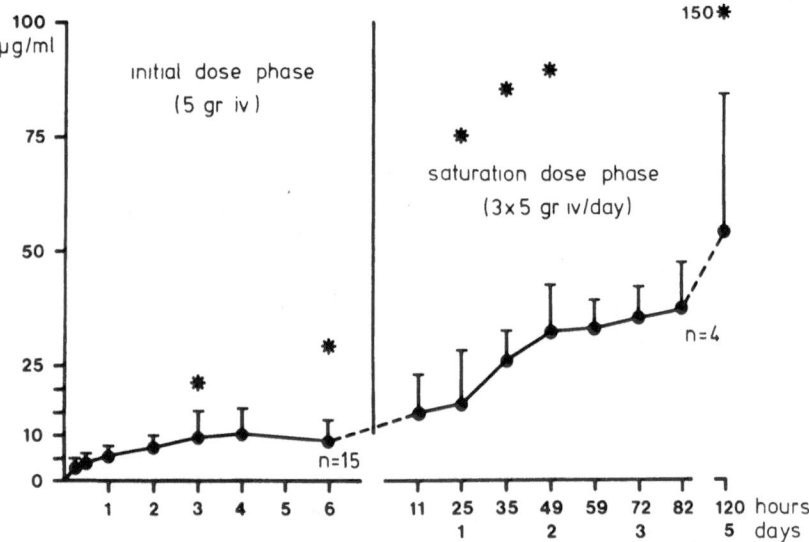

Fig. 2. Fosfomycin CSF penetration rate after continuous application of 5 g three times daily in the presence of an intact blood-brain barrier (mean values and standard deviation) (* single values of patients with inflamed meninges)

the CSF concentration curve was 39 µg/ml · h i.e. 9.24% of the AUC of the serum concentration curve.

Latency time could be markedly shortened with an initial dose of 10 g fosfomycin. Maximum values of 15.4 to 17.7 µg/ml were found between 120 and 360 minutes. The AUC for 10 g fosfomycin in the CSF concentration curve was nearly 14% (13.81%) of the corresponding serum AUC.

In further investigations a maintenance dose of 5 g three times daily was administered after an initial 5 g dose. The CSF concentration was observed continuously for 5 days and a marked saturation with fosfomycin in the CSF was seen (Fig. 2).

A mean CSF concentration of 32 µg/ml was achieved between the second and fifth day.

The CSF fluid from patients with bacterial meningitis who received fosfomycin for therapeutic reasons showed 100–250% higher concentrations of fosfomycin than the control group. This indicates a considerably increased CSF penetration in inflamed meninges.

Conclusion

Our investigations demonstrate that relevant concentrations of fosfomycin in the CSF can be established after an intravenous infusion of 5 g even when the blood brain barrier is intact. An increase of the dose from 5 to 10 g fosfomycin resulted in higher peak concentrations in a shorter time period. Total penetration lies between 9 and 14% of the administered dose as measured by the AUC.

We can confirm the findings of good liquor penetration of fosfomycin by others [1, 2]. Based upon a great number of patients and samples fosfomycin can thus be regarded as satisfactorily in penetrating the CSF both in the presence of an intact and disrupted blood brain barrier. The liquor penetration rate is significantly higher than that of penicillins, cephalosporines and aminoglycosides. This is explained by the favorable physico-chemical properties of the substance namely, the absence of protein binding, low molecular mass and small molecule size.

Clinical Experience

We have used fosfomycin in combination with other antibiotics in the treatment of postoperative or posttraumatic meningitis since 1982. Prophylactic administration of fosfomycin in the case of liquorrhea and after prolonged neurosurgical procedures has proven beneficial. Until now development of resistance of microorganisms has not been observed.

References

1. Ito H, Ikeda K, Kawano H, Kitasayashi M, Maeda M, Ishise J, Futami K, Yamamoto S (1982) Transfer of fosfomycin into cerebrospinal fluid. Jap J Antibiot 35: 2530–2534
2. Oellers B, Bethke RO, Fabricius K, Müller O (1981) Untersuchungen zur Liquorgängigkeit von Fosfomycin. Therapiewoche 31: 5855–5857
3. Vömel W, Abshagen U, Betzien G, Haag R, Hoffmann R (1981) Zur Humanpharmakokinetik und antibakteriellen In-vitro-Aktivität von Fosfomycin. Krankenhausarzt 54: 771–790

Author's address: Prof. Dr. G. Pfeifer, Universitätsklinik für Anästhesiologie, Sigmund-Freud-Strasse 25, D-5300 Bonn 1, Federal Republic of Germany.

Antimicrobial Therapy of Bacterial Meningitis in Premature- and Newborn Infants and Shunt Infections

J. P. Guggenbichler, G. Menardi, and J. Hager

Department of Pediatrics (Chairman: Prof. Dr. H. Berger),
Department of Surgery I (Chairman: Prof. Dr. F. Gschnitzer),
Division of Pediatric Surgery (Chairman: Prim. Dr. G. Menardi),
University of Innsbruck, Austria

Summary

Meningitis in premature and newborn infants due to gramnegative organisms is a serious disorder with high mortality and serious late sequelae. Also problems in the treatment of shunt infections were present in a great number of patients. Until a few years ago no uniformly accepted treatment modality for these life threatening disorders was available. Fosfomycin in combination with β lactam antibiotics and aminoglycosides has been intensively investigated in a theoretical and clinical study:

Bacteriological investigation: Numerous clinical isolates from premature and newborn infants with meningitis have been investigated for susceptibility to fosfomycin. All isolates were sensitive to fosfomycin with addition of 25 mg/l glucose-6-phosphate to the growth medium.

Animal studies: Fosfomycin was investigated in a lapine meningitis model. With a bolus injection of 100 mg/kg body weight and constant replacement of the eliminated amount of drug by an IV infusion the decrease in colony forming units was investigated in the CSF after cisternal puncture in three hourly intervals. Five of 6 strains were completely eliminated from the CSF within 6–9 hours. In one strain only a substantial reduction of the number of organisms in the CSF was observed.

Pharmacokinetic investigation: In the rabbit model and in infants the penetration of fosfomycin into the CSF was investigated. In the animal model where inflamed meninges were present, a penetration of fosfomycin into the CSF of 65% of concomitantly measured serum concentrations was seen. The penetration into the CSF in patients with not inflamed meninges at 3 hours was approximately 10% of concomitantly measured serum concentrations: after 8 hours CSF concentrations approached serum concentrations. In a therapeutic investigation in patients with inflamed meninges CSF concentrations of fosfomycin reached a plateau on day two to three in the therapeutic range.

In a comprehensive clinical investigation of meningitis in premature and newborn infants 36 patients have been treated with fosfomycin in combination with various β lactam antibiotics or aminoglycosides. The mortality was low, 1 patient died from a 3 × 4 cm measuring brain abscess 24 hours after initiation of fosfomycin therapy. 4 patients developed a hydrocephalus. Follow-up of 29 patients revealed recovery in 22, 5 patients are moderately retarded, two show severe psychomotor retardation.

In a further clinical study we investigated fosfomycin in the treatment of CSF infections in patients with infected ventriculo-atrial shunts. In the majority of these patients staphylococci have been isolated which can not be eliminated from the surface of silastic material by antibiotics alone. However, a 10 days treatment with fosfomycin plus oxacillin and gentamicin in combination with external drainage of the CSF into a closed system made it possible to exchange all parts of the system in one session without reinfection. This procedure was followed by the same antibiotic regimen postoperatively for 10–14 days. Under this treatment modality therapeutic results have been considerably better compared to previous treatment schedules.

Zusammenfassung

Die Behandlung der eitrigen Meningitis mit gramnegativen Enterobakterien bei Früh- und Neugeborenen war durch schlechte klinische Ergebnisse gekennzeichnet. Zum Teil besteht ein hohes Maß an Resistenz gegen die verwendeten Antibiotika (Aminopenicilline), teilweise penetrieren Antibiotika schlecht in den Liquorraum (Aminoglykoside) oder besitzen eine hohe Toxizität in diesem Lebensalter (Chloramphenicol, Trimethoprim). Fosfomycin ließ wegen des günstigen antimikrobiellen Wirkspektrums, der raschen bakteriziden Wirksamkeit, der synergistischen Wirkung mit verschiedenen β-Lactam-Antibiotika, der guten Liquorpenetration und der geringen Toxizität eine günstige Wirkung erwarten. Fosfomycin wurde daher in einer umfassenden theoretischen und klinischen Untersuchung in der Behandlung der eitrigen Meningitis bei Früh- und Neugeborenen untersucht.

In der weiteren Folge wurde außerdem aufgrund der günstigen Ergebnisse bei den theoretischen Untersuchungen auch eine klinische Untersuchung in der Behandlung von Shuntinfektionen durchgeführt.

Bakteriologische Untersuchung: Eine Reihe klinischer Isolate von Patienten mit eitriger Meningitis durch gramnegative Erreger wurde auf deren Empfindlichkeit auf Fosfomycin mit Zugabe von 25 mg/l Glukose-6-Phosphat im Nährmedium untersucht. Alle getesteten Keime waren auf Fosfomycin empfindlich. In einem Tiermodell (Kaninchenmodell nach M. Sande) wurde die Elimination verschiedener gramnegativer Erreger aus dem Liquorraum untersucht. 5 von 6 Keimen konnten aus dem Liquorraum innerhalb von 6—9 Stunden vollständig eliminiert werden. Beim 6. Stamm kam es zu einer substantiellen Keimreduktion.

Die Liquorpenetration wurde im Tiermodell bei entzündlich veränderten Meningen und beim Menschen im Rahmen einer pharmakokinetischen und therapeutischen Untersuchung bestimmt. Die Penetration von Fosfomycin beim Kaninchen betrug ca. 65% gleichzeitig gemessener Serumkonzentrationen. Beim Menschen betrugen die Konzentrationen von Fosfomycin in nicht entzündlich veränderten Meningen nach 3 Stunden ca. 10% der Serumkonzentration. Die dreimal tägliche Verabreichung führte zur Kumulation von Fosfomycin innerhalb von 24 bis 48 Stunden im Liquor und zu therapeutisch wirksamen Konzentrationen. Bei entzündlich veränderten Meningen werden am 2. bis 3. Behandlungstag Konzentrationen zwischen 25 und 40 µg/ml Liquor beobachtet.

In einer klinisch-therapeutischen Untersuchung wurde Fosfomycin bei 36 Patienten bisher in Kombination mit verschiedenen β-Lactam-Antibiotika oder Aminoglykosiden eingesetzt. Nur 1 Patient verstarb, bei 5 weiteren mußten Spätschäden beobachtet werden. 22 Patienten sind nun 1—6 Jahre nach Beendigung der Therapie psychomotorisch normal entwickelt.

Auch Infektionen beim ventilversorgten Hydrozephalus bereiten therapeutische Probleme. Ventilsysteme, die teilweise aus Plastikmaterial bestehen, können auf die Dauer nicht von festhaftenden Staphylokokkenplaques befreit werden. Entfernung dieses Fremdmaterials ohne ausreichende Liquorableitung kann eine lebensbedrohliche Zunahme des Hirndrucks hervorrufen, ein Austausch des Materials ohne vorherige Sanierung des Liquors behebt nicht die Infektion. Kombiniert man jedoch nach einem bestimmten Plan, der nach längeren klinischen Versuchen festgelegt wurde, bestimmte Antibiotika in parenteralen (Fosfomycin und Oxacillin) und intrathekalen (Gentamycin) Gaben mit einer externen Ableitung in ein geschlossenes System außerhalb des Körpers, so gelingt es zunächst, den Liquor zu sanieren und dann in einer Sitzung das gesamte System auszutauschen. Fosfomycin führt durch Kombination mit anderen

Antibiotika sowie dem Auswechseln der Shunt-Teile zu therapeutischen
Ergebnissen, die mit bisherigen Behandlungsmodalitäten nicht erreichbar
waren.

Introduction

Bacterial meningitis is a medical emergency and requires prompt
and appropriate antimicrobial chemotherapy. While therapeutic
results in bacterial meningitis in children over one month of age are
satisfactory with mortality rates between 1 and 3%, the treatment of
meningitis in premature and newborn infants, in children with
serious underlying disorders and with shunt infections is much less
successful. The mortality in this population ranges between 15 and
45% [1, 2].

Antimicrobial chemotherapy for these serious disorders faces
several problems:

An increase in resistance to aminopenicillins, standard therapy
for meningitis due to gramnegative enteric organisms in the last
years, has developed. Presently approximately 55% of isolates of E.
coli, 75% of Proteus spp. (indol positive and negative) and 95% of
Klebsiella Enterobacter in our clinic are resistant to this group of
antibiotics. Also, CSF cultures have remained positive for several
days despite of high CSF concentrations of the antibiotic.

Aminoglycosides do not reach adequate concentrations in the
CSF; the narrow therapeutic range of these antibiotics does not
permit an increase in the dosage due to the risk of systemic toxicity
[3].

Aminoglycosides also loose rapidly in antimicrobial activity with
decreasing pH. The pH in the CSF in bacterial meningitis is
frequently below 7.0.

Intralumbar administration of aminoglycosides does not allow
for an even distribution of the drug in the CSF, particularly in the
ventricular space and ventriculitis is a common (70%) complication
of gramnegative meningitis in newborn infants. A controlled
prospective randomized study showed no therapeutic advantage of
lumbar or intrathekal gentamicin plus systemic therapy over
systemic therapy alone [4].

Cotrimoxazol exhibits a favorable antimicrobial spectrum and good penetration into the CSF. In vitro 90% of E. coli isolates are presently susceptible to this combination of drugs in a ratio of 1 : 20 [5]. However, this favorable synergistic ratio has not been observed in vivo in the CSF. In a previous investigation from our institution a ratio of 1 : 3 was found. In addition there are problems with toxicity of this combination in premature and newborn infants: Sulfonamides replace bilirubin from albumin bindings sites and subject infants to the risk of kernikterus. Potential toxic effects of trimethoprim—an antimetabolite—on the growing brain has been postulated in newborn infants.

Chloramphenicol with its good penetration into the CSF and favorable inhibitory activity against gramnegative organisms has been used in the treatment of bacterial meningitis in neonates. This drug, however, works only bacteriostatically against enterobacteriae. Inhibition of the alternate pathway of complement by E. coli K_1, however, requires a bactericidal antibiotic to eradicate bacteria from the CSF [6]. In addition to its rare but serious side effects on the hematopoetic system it exhibits additional toxicity in the neonate. Due to the decreased rate of glucuronidation in the immature liver, toxic concentrations may accumulate, resulting in the potentially lethal "gray syndrome". Chloramphenicol should be used only when serum and CSF concentrations can be continuously monitored [7].

Cephalosporines I generation failed in clinical trials in the treatment of bacterial meningitis. During the last few years promising cephalosporines and azylureidopenicillins have been developed with markedly increased activity against gramnegative organisms. These drugs include cefotaxime, ceftriaxone, moxalactam, azlocillin und piperacillin. Excellent reduction in the number of viable organisms in the CSF has been observed in animal experiments. However, these newer agents are not uniformly successful clinically with slow eradication of bacterial organisms and recurrence of gramnegative meningitis [8].

Fosfomycin is a new antibiotic with a broad antimicrobial spectrum. Several reasons to consider fosfomycin alone or in combination with β-lactam antibiotics or aminoglycosides as alternative treatment of bacterial meningitis in high-risk neonates and children are:

1. Favorable antimicrobial activity against most organisms encountered in bacterial meningitis in premature and newborn infants and in shunt infections.

2. Small molecular weight and lack of protein binding allows good CSF and tissue penetration [9].

3. Low toxicity and broad therapeutic range.

Therefore this drug merits comprehensive theoretical and clinical investigation as to its applicability in the treatment of bacterial meningitis in these high risk patients.

Theoretical Investigations

Bacteriological Investigations

In vitro susceptibility studies were performed first.

Various isolates of bacterial meningitis from our institution and from the national meningitis study group were investigated by an agar dilution and a broth dilution method. Various concentrations of glucose-6-phosphate (ranging from 20 to 200 μg/ml) were added to the growth medium and MIC values were determined. These results were compared with susceptibility tests by measurements of zone diameters of 50 μg fosfomycin disks with addition of 25 and 200 μg glucose-6-phosphate/disk.

Table 1 shows the organisms investigated in the study and the results of MIC testing.

Animal Studies

The biological relevance of these MIC values with or without addition of glucose-6-phosphate was investigated in an animal model. This model was designed by M. Sande and allows the assessment of CSF penetration of various antibiotics, determination of their efficacy and the comparison of these new antibiotics with each other.

Table 1. Antimicrobial activity of fosfomycin against various organisms isolated from patients with bacterial meningitis

Organism	Number	MIC 50		MIC 100	
		With 25 mg/l Gluc. 6 PO_4	Without Gluc. 6 PO_4	With 25 mg/l Gluc. 6 PO_4	Without Gluc. 6 PO_4
E. coli	57	2	32	4	64
Salmonella	6	1	8	2	16
Citrobacter	6	1	4	4	16
Klebsiella	3	16	16	32	64
Proteus indol positive				1	4
Staphylococcus aureus	18	0.25	0.25	0.5	0.5
Streptococcus group B	6	0.5	0.5	1.0	1.0

Table 2. Number of colony forming units of various Enterobacteria in CSF after administration of 100 mg/kg body weight fosfomycin by IV bolus injection followed by IV infusion of 50 mg/kg body weight/h to New Zealand white rabbits

Organism	MIC values		Rabbit	Inoculum size	0 h	3 h	6 h	9 h
	With G6P	Without G6P						
C 47 E. coli	1	16	1	5×10^5	7×10^5	6×10^1	2×10^1	0
			2	2×10^4	5×10^4	2×10^3	3×10^2	4×10^1
			3	2×10^4	1×10^5	3×10^3	3×10^2	6×10^1
			4	1×10^5	6×10^4	2×10^3	4×10^2	0
			5	1×10^5	4×10^4	4×10^4	3×10^3	0
C 64 E. coli	4	32	1	1×10^6	2×10^3	5×10^3	5×10^3	1×10^1
			2	1×10^6	5×10^4	1×10^2	1×10^2	2×10^2
			3	5×10^5	5×10^3	2×10^3	—	—
C 58 E. coli	1	32	1	5×10^6	5×10^4	1×10^2	0	0
			2	5×10^6	5×10^4	1×10^2	0	0
			3	1×10^6	8×10^3	1×10^2	0	0
			4	1×10^6	8×10^3	1×10^2	0	0
C 72 E. coli	2	64	1	1×10^6	4×10^4	0	0	0
			2	1×10^6	1×10^6	2×10^1	2×10^1	0
			3	1×10^6	2×10^6	1×10^4	2×10^2	0
C 80 E. coli	1	4	1	1×10^5	8×10^6	5×10^2	1×10^1	0
			2	1×10^5	1×10^6	2×10^1	0	0
			3	5×10^5	5×10^5	2×10^2	0	0
			4	5×10^5	5×10^5	5×10^1	2×10^1	0
C 11 Citrobacter	4	4	1	5×10^5	4×10^5	3×10^2	2×10^1	0
			2	5×10^5	4×10^6	1×10^4	1×10^1	0

New Zealand white rabbits were prepared according to the method described by Sande and Dacey. $\sim 10^6$ organisms were inoculated intracisternally. 10–14 hours later a suboccipital puncture revealed signs of meningitis in the CSF (pleocytosis, elevation

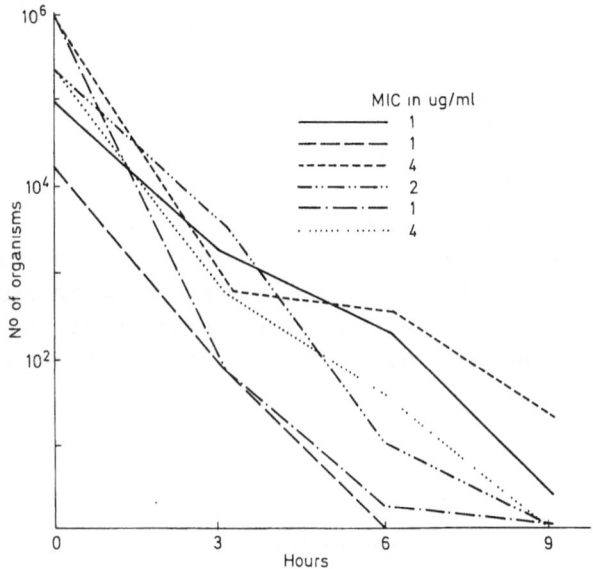

Fig. 1. Decrease in colony forming units over time periods

of protein, decrease of CSF sugar) and a mean of 5×10^5 viable organisms per ml CSF. Without treatment the number of organisms increased to 10^7 organisms/ml over the next 8 hours and the rabbits succumbed to the meningitis within 18 hours. Fosfomycin was given initially as an IV bolus injection of 100 mg/kg body weight followed by a continuous drip replacing the amount of drug lost by glomerular filtration. A constant serum concentration between 350 and 580 µg/ml was maintained. Fosfomycin concentrations in the CSF were determined and varied between 108 and 412 µg/ml (mean 285 µg/ml CSF). The penetration of fosfomycin into the CSF was at an average of 65% of concomitantly measured serum concentrations. The number of colony-forming units was determined in the CSF. Table 2 and Fig. 1 show elimination kinetics of bacterial organisms in the CSF in this rabbit model.

Results obtained in this rabbit model demonstrate that fosfomycin is capable of sterilizing the CSF within a short period of time in most instances. In comparison with data published by U. B. Schaad, elimination kinetics of bacteria under the influence of fosfomycin compare well with results obtained with gentamicin, ampicillin and moxalactam [10].

We realize that extrapoloation of these data to meningitis in humans must be done with great care, as this model differs in many ways from meningitis occurring in neonates (route of infection, production and circulation of the CSF in rabbits, natural resistance of rabbits to bloodstream infections etc.). Despite these drawbacks, the data encouraged us to proceed with a clinical investigation of fosfomycin in premature and newborn infants, in older children with meningitis due to gramnegative enteric organisms and shunt infections.

Clinical Investigations

Pharmacological Investigations

A pharmacokinetic investigation in newborn infants and older children preceeded the therapeutic trial. Fig. 2 shows a comparison of serum concentrations in newborn infants with 6-year-old children after administration of 25 mg fosfomycin per kg body weight. The pharmacokinetic parameters are described in an open one compartment model with first order invasion. Fosfomycin is excreted by the kidney with a halflife of approximately 1.5 hours in newborn infants and 1.0 hours in older children. The pharmacokinetics of fosfomycin are dose independent and doubling of the dose results in a linear increase of plasma concentrations. CSF concentrations of fosfomycin were determined after administration of 25 or 50 mg/kg body weight to newborn infants who received

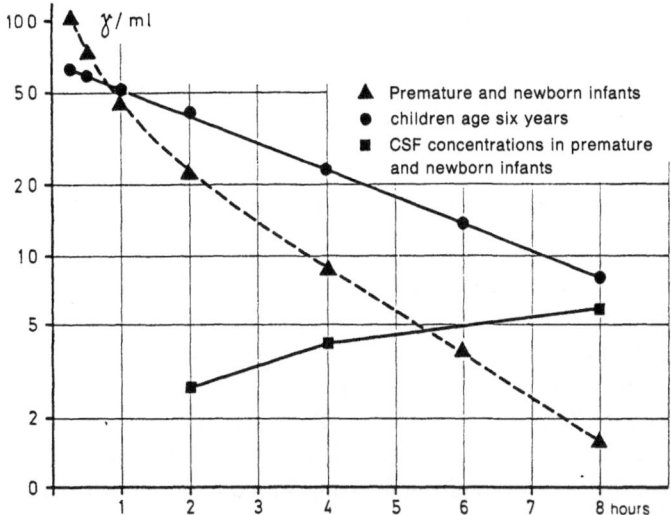

Fig. 2. Fosfomycin serum and CSF concentrations after IV bolus injection of 25 mg/kg body weight

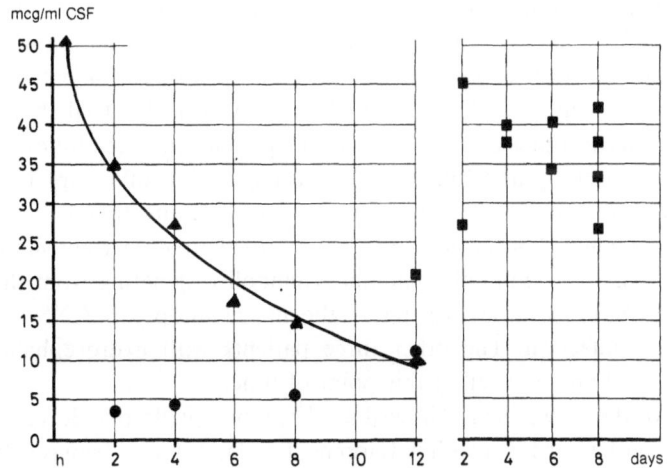

Fig. 3. Fosfomycin concentrations in serum ▲————▲ 25 mg/kg body weight. Fosfomycin concentrations in CSF after administration of ● 25 mg/kg body weight/8 h, ■ 50 mg/kg body weight/8 h in newborn infants

fosfomycin for treatment of suspected sepsis but without inflammatory changes in the CSF, when a routine lumbar puncture
was performed. Fig. 3 shows serum and CSF concentrations of
fosfomycin in 6 newborn infants.

Therapeutic Trials with Meningitis in Premature and Newborn Infants

36 premature and newborn infants with bacterial meningitis have
been treated between 1979 and 1986 in our institution with
fosfomycin 250 mg/kg body weight in three doses combined with a
β-lactam antibiotic (20) [azlocillin 150 mg/kg body weight (10),
ampicillin 200 mg/kg body weight (4), penicillin G (4) or cefotaxime
(2)], an aminoglycoside (gentamicin or tobramycin) 5 mg/kg body
weight (8) or chloramphenicol 30 mg/kg body weight (8). Table 3
shows the bacterial organisms isolated in the patients enrolled in the
therapeutic investigation.

Table 4 shows the immediate therapeutic outcome of these
patients treated in our institution.

There was one death in this group of patients: this patient died
within 24 hours after initiation of fosfomycin in combination with
cefotaxime from a brain abscess measuring 3 × 4 cm. 4 patients
suffer from hydrocephalus, treated with a ventriculo-atrial shunt.
The clinical course of 29 of 35 surviving patients has been followed
over the last 5 years; 4 patients have been lost for follow-up. Two
patients died in the meantime from reasons not directly related to
the meningitis. One of these two patients died after recurrent shunt
infections from multiple pulmonary emboli originating from the
distal ventriculo-atrial catheter. At the time of autopsy the CNS was
free of infection. The other three patients with hydrocephalus
recovered and are well at this point of time.

5 of these 29 patients showed a suboptimal intellectual development with retarded speech development and in IQ score between 75
and 90; two additional patients are severely retarded. 22 patients
developed normally. No motor disability or hearing defect was
observed.

Table 3. Bacterial organisms isolated from 36 patients with bacterial meningitis treated with Fosfomycin in various combinations

E. coli	16
Pseudomonas aeruginosa	3
Klebsiella	1
Proteus mirab.	1
Streptococcus group B	4
Streptococcus group A	1
Enterococci	1
Staphylococcus aureus	1
Pneumococci	1
Listeria monocytog.	1
Meningococci	1
No organism isolated pretreated with antibiotics	5
	36

Table 4. Therapeutic results in patients with bacterial meningitis treated with fosfomycin in various combinations (number of patients)

Immediate results	36
Death	1
Hydrocephalus	4
Recovered	31
Lost to follow-up	4
Death from unrelated reasons	2
Results of follow-up	29
Severely retarded	2
Moderately retarded	5
Well 1–6 years after treatment	22

Therapeutic Trial in Shunt Infections

Ventriculo-atrial shunt infections pose a formidable problem in pediatrics [11]. Since 1971 almost exclusively Holter valves were implanted with a ventriculo-atrial positioning. The implantation

Table 5. Bacterial organisms isolated in shunt infections

Organisms	Susceptible to			
	Total	Fosfomycin	Oxacillin	Gentamicin
Staphyloccus aureus	14	12	13	14
Staphylococcus albus	1	1	1	1
Pneumococcus	1	1	1	0
Enterococcus	1	1	0	1
Proteus mirab.	1	1	0	1
No organisms isolated	3			

itself and any further revision may lead to infection of the CSF and to a colonization of the valve.

Table 5 shows the organisms and their susceptibility isolated in our patients with shunt infections. Organisms most frequently encountered are staphylococci (coagulase positive and negative). These organisms elicit a comparatively low inflammatory response on the blood-brain barrier and hence a low penetration of β-lactam antibiotics into the CSF [12].

It proved to be extremely difficult to eradicate staphylococci colonizing silastic surfaces due to the formation of a mucoid barrier against penetration of β-lactam antibiotics [13]. Removal of the shunt system prior to eradication of the infecting organisms and insertion of a new system invariably results in reinfection. Removal of the infected shunt without establishing a ventricular drainage results in dangerous intracranial pressure elevation. The results of previous treatment modalities were unsatisfactory [11].

Our therapeutic approach consists of external drainage of the CSF in a closed system. Patients receive fosfomycin 250 mg/kg body weight in three doses in combination with oxacillin 160 mg/kg body weight divided into four to six doses. 2–5 mg of gentamicin L is

Table 6. Therapeutic regimen and treatment results of shunt infections

Phase I Treatment with fosfomycin in combination with oxacillin (2), rifampin (1), ceftriaxone (1). No exchange of the system.	4 patients	3 well, 1 death
Phase II Treatment with fosfomycin in combination with oxacillin, for 10–14 days, 2–5 mg gentamicin into Rickham reservoir 5 days. Removal of the infected shunt system and immediate implantation of a new system. Treatment with above-mentioned combination for 10–14 days.	9 patients	7 well, 2 deaths
Phase III Treatment with fosfomycin in combination with oxacillin 2–5 mg gentamicin L in Rickham reservoir.	6 patients	6 well
Or treatment with vancomycin in combination with oxacillin 2–5 mg gentamicin into Rickham reservoir. Simultaneous external drainage in a closed system for 10 days. Removal of the system and immediate implantation of a new system. Treatment with previous antibiotic regimen for 10–14 days.	2 patients	2 well

applied to the Rickham reservoir daily during the first 5 days. The choice of antibiotics depends on susceptibility testing: the majority of organisms were susceptible to fosfomycin and oxacillin; if organisms were resistant to either fosfomycin (2 of 18) or oxacillin (3 of 18) alternatives as vancomycin, ceftriaxone or rifampin were used. After an average of 10 days the whole system is removed and a new system implanted in the same session. This procedure is followed by the above-mentioned antibiotic regimen for 10–14 additional days.

Table 6 shows different modes of treatment and clinical outcome of our patients. In phase I (antimicrobial therapy alone without exchange of the system) one child out of four died. The use of antibiotics alone without exchange of the drainage system can be recommended only as a last resort if an operation can not be performed due to a critical clinical condition of the patient or if a further exchange of the system is impossible due to previous operations. This proceeding, however, bears a high risk of recurrence of infection.

In phase II we removed the infected system after treatment with antibiotics and replaced it immediately. Two patients died: one from shunt infection, a second from multiple pulmonary emboli originating on the distal catheter. Pulmonary emboli in this patient are possibly also related to infection. All patients in phase III are well. It is our conviction, that the combination of the abovementioned antibiotic regimen and a closed external drainage system is responsible for our therapeutic results which are clearly superior to data reported in the literature and to previous forms of treatment in our institution [12].

Conclusion

Fosfomycin has been investigated in bacteriologic, pharmacokinetic studies and in an animal model for its use in the treatment of bacterial meningitis in high-risk patients, i.e., premature and newborn infants and patients with shunt infections.

Results of therapeutic trials with fosfomycin in combination with various β-lactam antibiotics or aminoglycosides have been considerably better than the results obtained with previous therapeutic regimen without fosfomycin.

References

1. Kaplan S, Feigin R (1983) Treatment of bacterial meningitis in children. Ped Clin North Am 30: 259–269
2. Guggenbichler JP (1982) Behandlung der bakteriellen Meningitis im Kindesalter. Päd Pädol 17: 17–48
3. Strausbaugh L, Mandaleris CD, Sande MA (1977) Comparison of four aminoglycoside antibiotics in the therapy of experimental bacterial E. coli meningitis. J Lab Clin Med 89: 692–701

4. McCracken GH, Mize SG (1976) A controlled study of intrathekal antibiotic therapy in gramnegative enteric meningitis of infancy. Report of the neonatal meningitis cooperative study group. J Ped 89: 66–72

5. Sabel KG, Brandberg A (1975) Treatment of meningitis and septicemia in infancy with sulfamethoxazole-trimethoprim combination. Acta Pediatr Scand 34: 25–32

6. O'Toole RD, Thornton GF, Mukherjee MD (1976) Cerebrospinal immunoglobulins in bacterial meningitis; a possible role for antibody in penumococcal meningitis. Arch Neurol 25: 218–224

7. Goodman Gilman A, Goodman L, Gilman A (1980) The pharmacological basis of therapeutics, pp 1191–1199

8. Adler SP, Markowitz S (1983) Failure of moxalactam in the treatment of neonatal sepsis and meningitis from Salmonella typhimurium. J Ped 103: 913–916

9. Pfeiffer G (1986) Liquorspiegel von Fosfomycin und ihre klinische Relevanz. Symposium Fosfomycin-Arbeitstagung 1984, Hinterzarten, S 70–73

10. Schaad UB, McCracken GH, Loock CD, Thomas ML (1980) Pharmacokinetics and bacteriologic efficacy of moxalactam, cetotaxime, cetopetazone and R 13 9904 in experimental bacterial meningitis. Antimic Agents Chemoth 17: 406–410

11. Calleghan RP, Cohen SJ, Stewart GT (1961) Septicemia due to colonization of S/H valves by staphylococcus. Br Med J 64: 860–863

12. Frame PT, Mc Laurin RL (1984) Treatment of CSF shunt infection with intrashunt plus oral antibiotic therapy. J Neurosurg 60: 354–360

13. Peters G, Pulverer G (1985) Klinisch-mikrobiologische Aspekte und pathogenetische Grundlagen von „Plastik-Infektionen" durch Staphylokokken. Arzneimittelpraxis 15: 621–623

Authors' address: Doz. Dr. J. P. Guggenbichler, Universitäts-Kinderklinik, Anichstrasse 35, A-6020 Innsbruck, Austria.

Fosfomycin in Cerebral and Spinal Abscesses

H. Tritthart

Universitätsklinik für Neurochirurgie, Graz
(Vorstand: Prof. Dr. F. Heppner), Austria

Summary

The treatment of intracranial and spinal abscesses remains controversial. There are advocates for primary surgical excision, external drainage and/or antibiotic therapy. During the last four years 45 patients with intracranial and spinal abscesses were treated surgically with addition of fosfomycin therapy 2×8 g daily. Bacterial flora was sensitive to fosfomycin in only 31 of 45 patients (25 patients with intracranial, 6 patients with spinal abscesses) in whom fosfomycin treatment was continued postoperative; the other patients were treated with an antibiotic regimen according to the antibiogram.

Pharmakokinetic properties of fosfomycin were determined in these 31 patients and revealed excellent penetration of this agent into the brain abscess and its membrane. The bacteriologic cure rate was 96%. One patient with multiple brain abscesses expired in the immediate postoperative period. Two patients survived with severe neurological sequelae. No adverse side effects could be demonstrated by fosfomycin therapy. 8 g of fosfomycin given 12 hourly IV is highly effective in the treatment of abscesses in the CNS.

Zusammenfassung

Intrakranielle und spinale Abszesse sind mit einer hohen Mortalität und Morbidität verbunden. Gründe dafür liegen zum Teil auf seiten der Erkrankung: der oft unbekannten Ätiologie, den multipel resistenten Hospitalkeimen und in der Schwere des Verlaufs. Hirnabszesse entstehen entweder als fortgeleitete Infektion von einer Sinusitis oder Otitis media bzw. durch direkte Inokulation im Rahmen eines Traumas oder eines chirurgischen Eingriffes. Ein epiduraler spinaler Abszeß entsteht häufig auf der Basis einer Osteomyelitis eines Wirbelkörpers. Tuberkulöse Infektionen sind selten geworden.

Keime, die bei spinalen und intrakraniellen Abszessen isoliert werden, sind fakultativ anaerobe Streptokokken, Bakteroides spp, häufig werden jedoch koagulasepositive und -negative Staphylokokken sowie auch Enterobakterien gefunden. Zudem bestehen jedoch gravierende therapeutische Probleme.

Hier geht es um die Frage chirurgische Intervention allein, chirurgische Intervention + Antibiotika oder Antibiotika allein. Sowohl über den optimalen Operationszeitpunkt und die Operationstechnik als auch über die Wahl des Antibiotikums gibt es divergierende Meinungen.

β-Lactam-Antibiotika und Aminoglykoside besitzen eine schlechte Penetration in intrakranielle Abszesse und sind daher von unbefriedigenden therapeutischen Ergebnissen gefolgt.

Im Rahmen einer klinischen und pharmakokinetischen Untersuchung bei 45 Patienten mit intrakraniellen und spinalen Abszessen wurde Fosfomycin in Kombination mit chirurgischer Exzision des Abszesses untersucht. Von diesen ursprünglich 45 Patienten wurde bei 31 (25 Patienten mit intrakraniellen Abszessen, 6 mit spinalen Abszessen) ein fosfomycinempfindlicher Erreger isoliert und die Patienten entsprechend behandelt.

Die Patienten erhielten maximal 8 g Fosfomycin 2 × täglich oder je nach Körpergewicht weniger. Das Medikament wurde in jedem Fall gut vertragen, es wurden keine Nebenwirkungen beobachtet.

Im Rahmen einer pharmakokinetischen Untersuchung wurde bei 10 Patienten die Fosfomycinkonzentration in der Abszeßmembran und im Abszeßinhalt untersucht. Die Konzentrationen waren ähnlich hoch wie im Serum und betrugen im Mittel 170 µg/ml nach 120 Minuten.

Die ausgezeichnete Penetration von Fosfomycin ist neben der chirurgischen Intervention verantwortlich für die guten klinischen Ergebnisse. Nur 1 Patient von 31 verstarb an multiplen Hirnabszessen unmittelbar postoperativ. 2 Patienten zeigten wegen der ungünstigen Lokalisation des Herdes Spätschäden.

Patienten, die fosfomycinunempfindliche Keime im Abszess aufwiesen, wurden mit verschiedenen anderen Antibiotika (Cephalosporine, Aminoglykoside) behandelt. 4 dieser 14 Patienten verstarben.

Bei allen Patienten mit spinalen Abszessen konnte eine bakteriologische Heilung, bei 5 eine klinische Heilung erzielt werden.

Zusammenfassend kann festgestellt werden, daß ausgezeichnete Behandlungsergebnisse bei intrakraniellen und intraspinalen Abszessen mit Fosfomycin und Exzision des Abszesses zu erzielen sind, was einerseits auf der guten antimikrobiellen Wirksamkeit von Fosfomycin auf die isolierten Keime als auch auf der guten Penetration des Präparates in den Abszeßherd beruht.

Introduction

Despite of advances in neurosurgical operation techniques, neuroradiological investigation methods and the introduction of many potent antibiotics the morbidity and mortality of brain abscesses is still high [1, 2, 3]. This may be due to the in many cases still unknown mechanisms of origin and course of this disease as well as to divergent views concerning the nature, time and necsssity of surgery [4]. The situation is further complicated by difficulties in detecting and culturing the bacteria causing the disease and by special features of the blood-brain barrier with the necessity of CSF penetration of the chemotherapeutic agents. Similar problems are apparent in spinal abscesses which occur more rarely than brain abscesses [5]. This clinical picture is characterized less by high mortality than by a considerably morbidity. Infection transmitted from osteomyelitis of vertebral bodies is generally identified as the most frequent reason for epidural abscesses of the spinal canal, whereas the rare subdural empyema almost always arises hematogenically. Tuberculous inflammation of the spinal canal which predominated in previous years has been displaced today by staphylococcal infections.

Brain abscesses are frequently caused by transmission from infections such as chronic sinusitis, otitis media or by direct inoculation of organisms by trauma or surgery. In addition brain abscesses may also be caused by metastatic infections as in bacterial endocarditis. Congenital cardiac malformations and chronic lung conditions have lost significance as the underlying cause of abscesses. In these cases hypoxia may have caused circumscribed brain lesions and thus promoted bacterial colonization at the site of reduced resistance.

Until a few years ago baceriological analyses of brain abscesses revealed no organisms in about 50% of the cases. There has been a major change in this respect owing to improved bacteriological isolation techniques and the possibility of culturing anaerobic bacteria. Various studies have established streptococci, staphylococci, Bacteroides spp. and enterobacteria (e.g. enterobacter) as the most frequent organisms isolated from brain abscesses [1, 4]. Some of these bacteria are either obligatory or facultative anaerobes and may have previously escaped isolation. In staphylococcal infections enzymatic inactivation of antibiotics (e.g. penicillin) poses an additional problem. In our patients this has gained importance in view of the increased occurrence of staphylococcal infections. In order to treat this wide spectrum of bacteria effectively bactericidal and bacteriostatic antibiotics have been combined although antagonism of the employed drugs may occur in these treatment regimen. Consequently the therapeutic outcome frequently was unsatisfactory. This gap appears to have been filled by the introduction of fosfomycin.

Pharmacokinetic and Clinical Investigation

We report on 45 patients with cerebral and spinal abscesses who were treated in the last four years at the Neurosurgery division, Graz University Medical School. There were 39 patients with brain abscess and 6 patients with spinal abscesses (Table 1).

The average age of the male patients with brain abscesses was 37.5 years (minimum 2, maximum 67 years) and 40.7 years (minimum 16, maximum 59 years) for females.

Injuries were the most frequent cause of infection. In 20.5% of patients the etiology of the brain abscess was undetermined (Table 2). The localization of the brain abscesses depended on their etiology: in our patients they were most frequently found in the temporal lobe. There were 3 patients with multiple abscesses (7.69%) and no case with abscesses in the cerebellum was seen (Table 3).

Table 1. Cerebral and spinal abscesses (1981–1984)

Male	37.5 years	(2 a minimum – 67 a maximum)
Female	40.7 years	(16 a minimum – 59 a maximum)

Table 2. Cerebral abscesses (1981–1984)

Etiology

Source of infection	Number of patients (%)
Ear	7 (18)
Frontal sinus	3 (7.6)
Trauma	10 (25.7)
Blood	5 (12.8)
Surgery	6 (15.4)
Unknown	8 (20.5)
	39 (100)

Table 3. Cerebral abscesses (1981–1984)

Location	Number of patients (%)
Frontal lobe	9 (23.1)
Temporal lobe	17 (43.7)
Parietal lobe	7 (18)
Occipital lobe	3 (7.6)
Multiple	3 (7.6)
	39 (100)

Symptoms of the brain abscesses included elevation of intracranial pressure and focal neurological deficits. Both spinal and cerebral abscesses were verified by axial computerized tomography combined with myelography in patients with spinal processes.

Depending on the clinical presentation and the results of the radiological investigation the brain abscess was either drained, extirpated or, when a diffuse infiltration was present, suppuration under antibiotic protection was awaited as long as the clinical condition of the patient permitted. Bacteriological investigations

Table 4. Bacteriology of brain abscesses (1981–1984)

Organisms		Number of patients
Streptococcus		7
aerobic	5	
anaerobic	2	
Haemophilus inf.		4
Staphylococcus		16
S. aureus	11	
S. epidermidis	5	
Escherichia coli		3
Bacteroides		4
Pseudomonas		2
Enterobacter sp.		2
Fusobacterium nucleatum		1
		39

Table 5. Bacteriology of brain abscesses treated with fosfomycin
(1981–1984)

Organisms		Number of patients
Staphylococcus		16
S. aureus	11	
S. epidermidis	5	
Haemophilus inf.		4
Escherichia coli		3
Bacteroides		2
		25

were performed and consisted of aerobic and anaerobic cultures (Table 4).

31 of 45 isolates were sensitive to fosfomycin (Table 5). These patients (25 with cerebral, 6 with spinal abscesses) received fosfomy-

Table 6. Brain abscesses treated with fosfomycin (1981–1984)

Organisms		
Staphylococcus	16	monotherapy
S. aureus	11	
S. epidermidis	5	
Escherichia coli	3	monotherapy
Haemophilus inf.	4	moxalactam
Bacteroides	2	cefoxitin

Table 7. Fosfomycin concentration in serum and brain abscess (pus) and abscess membran. 2×8 g IV BID (N = 10)

t/min	Serum µg/ml	Pus µg/ml	Membrane µg/g
30	420 ± 53		
60	380 ± 36		
120	125 ± 28	171 ± 12	112 ± 29
360	43 ± 11		

cin postoperatively for an average of 14 days. Depending on the bacteria, fosfomycin was administered as mono- or as combination therapy (Table 6). Patients received a maximum of 2×8 g of fosfomycin daily via a central venous catheter or less according to their body weight. The 14 patients with abscesses caused by bacteria not sensitive to fosfomycin received an antibiotic regimen adjusted in accordance to the antibiogram. In all patients also one of the above-mentioned surgical procedures was performed.

Fosfomycin concentration in pus and in the abscess capsule was examined in 10 patients with brain abscess caused by fosfomycin sensitive bacteria (Table 7). Analysis revealed excellent penetration of the drug into the inflamed parts of the brain in some cases equalling the concentration found in serum. The highest concentrations were found in circumscribed areas of inflammation without a solid capsule. However, adequate concentrations were also found both in the abscess membrane and in pus.

Due to high concentrations of active drug in the abscess membrane and its contents the results of fosfomycin treatment at our hospital were excellent and were followed by elimination of bacteria. No allergic reactions, gastrointestinal symptoms, significant alterations on blood tests (e.g. clotting studies) or other side effects resulting from fosfomycin therapy were observed.

One patient with multiple abscesses and ventricular infiltration died in the immediate postoperative period. In two patients a permanent neurological deficit was unavoidable due to the location of the abscess. Consecutive hydrocephalus has not yet been detected in any of these patients and the period of observation is too short to decide whether epileptic attacks will be caused by abscesses.

All of the spinal processes were due to staphylococci and bacterial clearance with fosfomycin was achieved in every patient. Recovery from this disease depended on the preoperative state of the patient. In one patient spastic diplegia present before operation was not improved but in five other cases the neurological deficit has largely regressed and patients are able to walk again.

Discussion

Intracranial and spinal abscesses are associated with a high mortality and morbidity. Out of 39 patients with brain abscesses 25 were treated with fosfomycin in accordance with the antibiogram. In this patient group 1 patient died. In the 14 patients with brain abscesses not suitable for fosfomycin therapy (bacterial spectrum insensitive to fosfomycin) four patients died. In the patient group which could be treated with fosfomycin the high rate of bacterial clearance was striking. This may be due to the small molecular mass and high CSF penetration of the drug, demonstrated by high concentrations of fosfomycin in the abscess membrane and pus. Antibiotic treatment in this group lasted up to 20 days postoperatively and no inflammatory relaps was observed. Unfavorable recovery chances in the presence of bacteria unresponsive to fosfomycin and chloramphenicol is often due to the poor CSF penetration of alternative antibiotics such as cephalosporines and aminoglycosides. Our investigations confirm that abscesses of the central nervous system must still be regarded as potentially fatal diseases. Cure depends on the possibility of surgical intervention and the efficacy of antibiotic treatment. Especially for penicillin resistant staphylococcal infections of the central nervous system fosfomycin has proved to be an excellent and highly effective antibiotic and can be recommended as monotherapy after surgical extirpation of the focus of inflammation.

References

1. Yang S-Y (1981) Brain abscess: a review of 400 cases. J Neurosurg 55: 794–799
2. Fischer EG, McLennan JE, Suzuki Y (1981) Cerebral abscess in children. Am J Dis Child 135: 746–749
3. George B, Roux F, Pillon M, Thurel C, George C (1979) Relevance of antibiotics in the treatment of brain abscesses. Acta Neurochirurgica 47: 285–291
4. Haley EC, Costello GT, Rodeheaver GT, Winn HR, Scheld WM (1983) Treatment of experimental brain abscess with penicillin and chloramphenicol. J Infect Dis 148: 737–744
5. Messer HD, Lenchner GS, Brust JCM, Resor S (1977) Lumbar spinal abscess managed conservatively. J Neurosurg 46: 825–829

Author's address: Dr. H. Tritthart, Universitätsklinik für Neurochirurgie, Auenbruggerplatz, A-8036 Graz, Austria.

Fosfomycin in the Treatment of Chronic Osteitis

B. Roth, G. Mattarelli, and F. Bartels

Chirurgische Klinik, Bezirksspital Wattenwil, Wattenwil, Switzerland

Summary

55 patients suffering from chronic posttraumatic or postsurgical osteitis were treated by surgical intervention and antimicrobial therapy with fosfomycin. All patients have undergone one or more conventional treatment trials (surgical clensing, immobilization, antiseptics) before. At the time of this combined therapeutic approach the disease had lasted a mean of 3.3 years (maximum 8 years). Postoperatively the first group of 28 patients was treated with 5 g fosfomycin twice daily as intravenous infusion in addition to the above mentioned surgical treatment. Since fosfomycin showed no serious side-effects (1 × phlebitis, 1 × diarrhea) the second group of patients was treated with a daily intravenous dose of 15 g fosfomycin. The treatment with fosfomycin was administered for a mean of 14 days (range 8–21 days). At the end of treatment the drainage fluid was sterile in 49 patients (88%). Remarkable was the early appearance of granulation tissue and fast healing of wounds in patients treated with fosfomycin. During the 18 month follow-up 8 patients developed a relapse. Although this short period of observation does not imply a final conclusion, it should be emphasized, that the results of this therapeutic regimen are exceedingly better than the results seen in similar patient groups who received no fosfomycin.

Zusammenfassung

Die chronisch rezidivierende posttraumatische oder postoperative Osteitis ist eine gefürchtete Komplikation mit unbefriedigenden Behandlungsergebnissen. Willenegger führte 1962 die radikale chirurgische Herdsanierung mit Saug-Spül-Drainage in die Behandlung ein. In jüngerer Zeit wurde zusätzlich zur chirurgischen Behandlung die Implantation von Aminoglykosid-Ketten (Palakos) oder die lokale Behandlung mit Antiseptika empfohlen. Dieses Konzept wird gegenwärtig von der Arbeitsgemeinschaft für Osteosynthese allgemein anerkannt.

Hier wird über die Behandlungsergebnisse von 55 Patienten, die zusätzlich zur chirurgischen Behandlung Fosfomycin 2 × 5 g, später 3 × 5 g täglich erhielten, berichtet. Alle Patienten wurden bereits mehrfach vorher erfolglos mit den gängien Behandlungsschemata behandelt. Die Krankheitsdauer vor Beginn der Fosfomycintherapie betrug im Mittel 3,3 Jahre. Die Keime, die präoperativ isoliert wurden, waren überwiegend multipel resistente Hospitalkeime; bei ⅔ der Patienten wurden Mischinfektionen mit mehreren Keimen beobachtet.

Nach einer Behandlungsdauer von im Durchschnitt 14 Tagen waren bei 49 Patienten die Kulturen steril. Bei 5 Patienten konnte innerhalb von 3 Wochen kein therapeutischer Erfolg erzielt werden. Bemerkenswert war jedoch die rasche Bildung von Granulationsgewebe, aber auch die perioperative Blutungsneigung — ein erwünschter Befund — in der Knochenchirurgie —, die jedoch nicht auf pathologischen Gerinnungsparametern beruhte.

Bei 7 Patienten (12,7%) wurde innerhalb einer Beobachtungszeit von 18 Monaten ein Rezidiv diagnostiziert. Gleichzeitig wurde jedoch bei Patienten unter Behandlungsschemata ohne Fosfomycin eine Rezidivrate im Bereich von 24% beobachtet.

Obwohl die Nachbeobachtung von 18 Monaten relativ kurz ist, kann dennoch festgestellt werden, daß die unmittelbaren Behandlungsergebnisse des Behandlungsschemas mit Fosfomycin günstig sind und eine bemerkenswert niedrige Rate an Rezidiven zu beobachten ist.

Introduction

Chronic posttraumatic or postoperative osteitis is still one of the most feared complications of bone surgery. Irrigation-suction drainage introduced in 1962 by Willenegger was generally regarded as a valid concept for treatment for many years.

Recently alternatives to the classical technique have arisen. These include the gentamycin-Palakos beads introduced by Klemm in 1972 and the treatment of chronic osteitis with local antiseptics as propagated by Müller in 1980. This latter concept is regarded by most hospitals of the Arbeitsgemeinschaft für Osteosynthese (Working group on Osteosynthesis) as binding.

Clinical Investigation

We present a report of 55 patients with chronic postoperative osteitis who were treated with fosfomycin in combination with the usual surgical and antiseptic therapy. These patients had been treated repeatedly before according to current valid therapeutic regimen with precise surgical cleansing of the focus of infection, immobilization and antiseptic treatment without success. All the patients suffered relapses requiring renewed surgical therapy and were treated additionally at this time with fosfomycin. The case histories of these patients are strikingly long-lasting with an average of 3.3 years and a maximum of 8 years. All 55 patients had undergone between 2 and 21 prior surgical cleansing operations because of generally fistulating relapses.

Site of the infectious process: 25 of these patients suffered from posttraumatic osteitis of the tibia, 12 from infection of the thigh, 3 from infection in the metatarsus, 2 from infection in the radius. 11 bone infections followed endoprosthetic operations of the hip, 2 bone infections appeared in the iliac creast after removal of spongiosa. Preoperative bacteriologic investigations were carried out routinely before starting fosfomycin therapy. It is remarkable that most of the organisms are multiple resistant hospital acquired organisms. Mixed infections with 2–4 different pathogens were present in 41 of the 55 patients. Only 14 patients were infected with a single pathogen 13 of them with staphylococcus aureus hemolyticus.

Table 1 shows the organisms isolated preoperatively:

Table 1

Staphyloccus aureus	41
Enterococci	22
Pseudomonas aeruginosa	20
E. coli	15
Proteus mirabilis	14
Klebsiella spp.	9
Serratia	6
Citrobacter	3

40 patients were treated preoperatively once, 15 patients twice
with 5 g of fosfomycin in an IV infusion. Postoperatively an initial
group of 28 patients was treated with 2 × 5 g fosfomycin daily IV in
addition to the standard therapy mentioned above. No side effects
from fosfomycin therapy were observed in this group of patients.
Relapses during treatment led us to increase the dosage to 3 × 5 g
daily in a second group of 27 patients. In this group 3 patients
showed gastrointestinal side effects (diarrhea) with no therapeutic
consequences.

We do not intend to go into further detail of surgical management of bone infections in this report. We only wish to mention that
all clensed sites were either drained with Redon-Drains or broad
wound excision was performed. Bacteriological examination of
drains in situ or secretions from open foci was done routinely on the
7th, 14th and 21st postoperative day.

Table 2. Postoperative bacteriological monitoring

Cultures negative on	Number of patients
Day 7	24
Day 14	44
Day 21	50

These data indicate, that 5 patients did not prove bacteriologi-
cally sterile even after 21 days. The osteitis did not subside in any of
these 5 patients during the further course of treatment. We can
therefore conclude that the surgical clensing operation alone is
inadequate and the therapeutic success in the other patients comes
from the combination of surgery with antimicrobial therapy with
fosfomycin.

Fosfomycin therapy was terminated as soon as the bacteriological test proved negative, usually after 14 days. In cases remaining

Table 3. Duration of therapy

Up to 7 days	11 patients
Up to 14 days	32 patients
Up to 21 days	12 patients
(Average 14.2 days)	

positive over 3 weeks fosfomycin therapy should be terminated and renewed extensive surgical clensing performed.

Patients treated with fosfomycin showed a strikingly rapid formation of clean granulation tissue. We observed that the pits left by focus excision were generally filled completely with fine granulation tissue within 7–14 days. The phenomenon responsible for this exceedingly rapid granulation time is still not explicable. Patients undergoing fosfomycin therapy also bled considerably more during the operation, a desirable effect in osteitis therapy. Further laboratory investigations of hemostasis did not reveal any pathological clotting parameters in contrast to the phenomenon known as cephalosporine bleeding. Perhaps the small mass of the fosfomycin molecule improves microcirculation in some yet unknown way.

Treatment of these 55 patients was completed 18 months ago and follow-up examinations showed only 7 clinical relapses (12.7%). Since there is general agreement that chronic osteitis can only be brought to a standstill but can't be cured we fully realize that this short observation period does not permit a final conclusion. 5 of these relapses were single pathogen, 2 were mixed pathogen infections; Staphyloccus was isolated 5 times, Pseudomonas aeruginosa in 3 instances, Serratia and enterococci once each.

In comparison patients treated in our hospital with the same surgical operation technique with antiseptics but without fosfomycin during the same time period show an average relaps rate of 24%. However, most of the patients of this purely antiseptic group were being treated for the first time and so cant be compared fairly to the group where fosfomycin was employed.

Conclusion

We may conclude that precise surgical clensing in combination with fosfomycin therapy is highly successful therapy for posttraumatic or postoperative osteitis and has effected a clear decrease in the number of relapses as compared to modes of therapy without addition of fosfomycin.

Authors' address: Doz. Dr. B. Roth, Chirurgische Klinik, Bezirksspital Wattenwil, CH-3135 Wattenwil, Switzerland.

Resistance of Intracellular Killing of Staphylococci by Macrophages as New Pathophysiologic Concept of Acute Hematogenous Osteomyelitis in Children and Therapeutic Consequences

J. P. Guggenbichler, H. Bonatti, and *F. Rottensteiner*

Universitäts-Kinderklinik, Innsbruck (Chairman: Prof. Dr. H. Berger), Austria

Summary

The pathophysiologic mechanisms of acute hematogenous osteomyelitis in children has been investigated before. The unique blood supply of the metaphyseal marrow cavity with turbulent blood flow present in dilated sinusoid venoles contributes largely to bacterial adherence and abscess formation of bacteria in this area of bone. No clues, however, are provided as to why staphylococci are the most prevalent organisms isolated in this disorder. Investigations on phagocytosis and intracellular killing of bacteria in granulocytes under fluctuating concentrations in various antibiotics in a kinetic model revealed, that certain strains of staphylococcus aureus are able to resist killing after phagocytosis, β lactam antibiotics with poor penetration into phagocytes are unable to eradicate these intracellular surviving organisms. Fosfomycin, clindamycin and various combinations of these antibiotics with β lactam antibiotics and among each other show a synergistic mode of action in broth and broth + addition of serum and granulocytes and are also able to eradicate these intracellularly surviving staphylococci.

In a clinical study with 30 patients conservative treatment of acute hematogenous osteomyelitis in children has been attempted with an initial combination of a β lactam antibiotic (cefamandole or oxacillin) with fosfomycin followed after a mean of 10.5 days by oral clindamycin. The overall therapeutic success was excellent. 29 children were cured, in one patient therapy was discontinued due to a questionable bone marrow depression. One patient showed a radiologic, but not functional bone defect of the calcaneus.

We conclude from these findings:

The pathophysiologic mechanism of acute hematogenous osteomyelitis could be extended: Staphylococci invade the bloodstream of infants and children. The unique blood supply in the metaphyseal marrow cavity facilitates the organisms to be taken up by phagocytes. Certain strains of Staphylococcus aureus, however, are able to resist intracellular killing by macrophages and granulocytes. Surviving bacteria eventually kill the phagocyte thereby releasing more bacteria. Eventually an abscess forms. Fosfomycin and clindamycin and various combinations of these antibiotics but not β lactam antibiotics alone are able to eradicate intracellular staphylococci.

This theoretical concept was proven by a successful clinical trial in patients with hematogenous osteomyelitis.

Zusammenfassung

Untersuchungen des pathogenetischen Mechanismus der akuten hämatogenen Osteomyelitis zeigten, daß Besonderheiten in der Blutversorgung der epiphysennahen Diaphysenenden, insbesondere langer Röhrenknochen, das Angehen einer Infektion erleichtern. In großen sinusoiden Venolen ist der Blutstrom turbulent und erleichtert bakteriellen Mikroorganismen das Eindringen in das Knochenmark. Dieses Konzept gibt jedoch keinen Aufschluß darüber, warum gerade Staphylokokken am häufigsten als Erreger der akuten hämatogenen Osteomyelitis gefunden werden. Untersuchungen der Absterbekinetik von Keimen in Gegenwart von Frischplasma und Granulozyten/Makrophagen unter fluktuierenden Konzentrationen verschiedener Antibiotika zeigten, daß bestimmte Staphylokokkenstämme nach deren Phagozytose über zahlreiche Stunden in phagozytären Vakuolen überleben können. Durch die Bildung von z. B. Leukozidinen sind Staphylokokken imstande, die Bildung von H_2O_2, einen wesentlichen Schritt in der intrazellulären Abtötung von Keimen, zu blockieren. β-Laktam-Antibiotika, die praktisch nicht in Phagozyten penetrieren, können diese intrazellulär überlebenden Staphylokokken nicht eliminieren. Fosfomycin und Clindamycin bzw. verschiedene Kombinationen dieser beiden Antibiotika mit β-Laktam-Antibiotika und untereinander zeigen einerseits eine synergistische bakterizide Wirkung auf Staphylokokken extrazellulär und sind auch imstande, phagozytierte Staphylokokken in phagozytischen Vakuolen abzutöten.

Diese Befunde erlauben uns, unsere pathophysiologischen Vorstellun-

gen bezüglich der akuten hämatogenen Osteomyelitis zu erweitern: Staphylokokken dringen in die Blutbahn ein, werden aufgrund der Besonderheiten
der Blutversorgung der epiphysennahen Diaphysenden der Knochen
bevorzugt von Makrophagen und Granulozyten im Knochenmark phagozytiert. Bestimmte Stämme sind jedoch imstande, intrazellulär nach
Phagozytose zu überleben bzw. sich sogar zu vermehren und den Makrophagen zu töten; damit werden weitere Keime freigesetzt. Letztlich entsteht
ein Markabszeß, der sich in die Kompakta und subperiostal ausbreitet. β-
Laktam-Antibiotika allein können jedoch die intrazellulär überlebenden
Keime nicht eliminieren.
    Dieses Konzept wurde in einer klinischen Untersuchung bei 30 Patienten überprüft. Diese Patienten wurden ausschließlich konservativ mit einer
Kombination von Fosfomycin mit einem β-Laktam-Antibiotikum initial
intravenös behandelt; nach im Mittel 10,5 Tagen (4—14 Tagen) wurde die
Behandlung mit Clindamycin über weitere 3—8 Wochen oral fortgesetzt.
Die Behandlungsergebnisse waren ausgezeichnet. 29 Patienten konnten
klinisch geheilt werden, bei einem Patienten bestand ein radiologischer
Defekt des Kalkaneus, der jedoch keine funktionellen Störungen nach sich
zog. Bei einer Patientin mußte Fosfomycin wegen einer fraglichen Knochenmarkdepression vorzeitig abgesetzt werden.

Introduction

Osseous infections occur by three mechanisms:
    1. Acute hematogenous seeding following septicemia or
bacteremia.
    2. Direct inoculation of bone by a puncture wound or open
fracture.
    3. Contiguous spread from an adjacent focus of infection [1].
    In children most bone infections are hematogenous in origin and
frequently involve the metaphysis. Any of the pyogenic organisms
may be responsible for osteomyelitis; in the vast majority of
instances the offending organisms are staphylococci, especially in
children under 2 years of age [2].
    There is still some controversy about the pathomechanisms
responsible for hematogenous osteomyelitis: Most of these infections begin in the metaphyseal marrow cavity, presumably
because this is the most richly vacularized portion of the bone and

therefore most exposed to blood-borne organisms. Organisms that reach the metaphyseal area lodge in the region of the vascular loops; end arteries that feed the loops continue directly into the capillaries which in turn empty into relatively dilated venous channels. Here the blood flow is turbulent and slow. It has been postulated that these conditions favor minute vascular occlusions and are supportive to bacterial adherence, growth and abscess formation. This theory, however, does not provide any clues as to why staphylococci are the most frequent organisms isolated in this disorder [3].

Previous investigations of phagocytosis and intracellular killing of bacteria under fluctuating concentrations of antibiotics in a model recently developed in our institution indicated that certain strains of Staphylococcus aureus isolated from patients with acute hematogenous osteomyelitis are resistant to intracellular killing after phagocytosis. It was of interest to investigate this mechanism further and to apply the results to a rational therapy of hematogenous osteomyelitis.

Material and Methods

Theoretical Investigations

Model

A vessel filled with 3,000 ml of a sterile glucose electrolyte solution identical in composition and osmotic pressure with Müller-Hinton broth (compartment I) was held at a constant temperature of 37 °C. A smaller chamber with a capacity of 8 ml (compartment II) oscillated in this vessel. This chamber was separated from compartment I by a dialysis membrane with a pore size of 1 nm. Compartment II was filled with Müller-Hinton broth and bacteria; in various experiments human granulocytes with and without fresh human plasma were added. The granulocytes were prepared by methods previously described [4]. Bacteria and granulocytes were incubated in these experiments for 8 hours at 37 °C.

Various antibiotics were added to compartment II: according to a concentration gradient the antibiotics were allowed to diffuse into compartment I with a halflife similar to that observed in vivo (usually 1.5 hours). 0.2 ml samples were taken every hour from compartment II for determination of antibiotic concentrations and colony forming units. Granulocyte preparations were observed in a darkfield microscope for phagocytosis of bacteria and documented by photography.

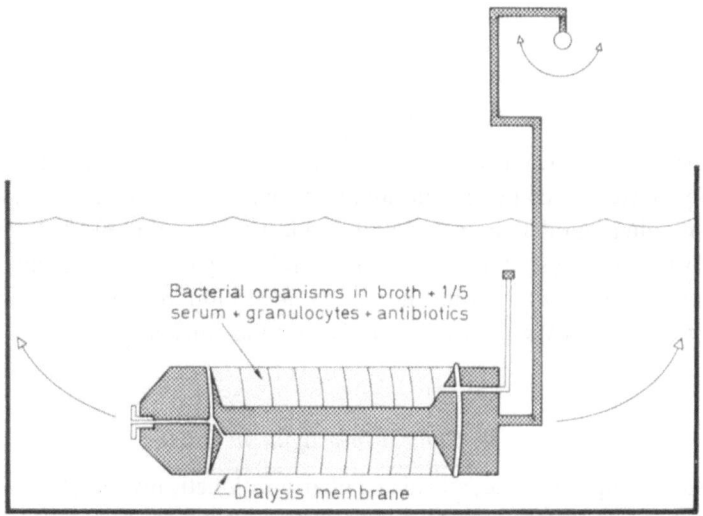

Fig. 1. Diagram of the kinetic model used for investigation of kill kinetics of staphylococci under fluctuating concentrations of various antibiotics

At the end of the 8-hour experiment, granulocytes were separated from surviving bacteria in the broth by several centrifugation and filtration steps. Granulocytes were harvested, disrupted by osmotic lysis and the number of viable organisms within the granulocytes was determined.

Fig. 1 shows a diagram of this model.

Kill kinetics and regrowth pattern of various bacteria in broth were investigated in this model [5]. In this publication we describe kill kinetics of a clinical isolate of Staphylococcus aureus from a blood culture of a patient with acute hematogenous osteomyelitis in broth and in broth + plasma + phagocytes under the influence of fluctuating concentrations of cefamandole (50 µg/ml peak concentration), fosfomycin (50 µg/ml peak concentration), Clindamycin (25 µg/ml peak concentration) and various combinations of these antibiotics. In this study we also investigated the influence of these antibiotics on metabolic properties of this organism, e.g., hemolysis of red blood cells and fibrinogen activation.

Pharmacokinetic Investigation

Prior to a clinical investigation serum and tissue concentrations of fosfomycin in compact bone and bone marrow were determined in an animal model and in man [6]. Table 1 shows concentrations of fosfomycin in serum, bone marrow and compact bone in animals and in man after intravenous administration of 100 mg/kg or 75 mg/kg body weight respectively as bolus injection.

Clinical Investigations

According to our theoretical and pharmacokinetic investigations 30 patients with acute hematogenous osteomyelitis have been treated initially during the last 5 years with a combination of a β lactam antibiotic (oxacillin or cefamandole) and fosfomycin. 250 mg/kg body weight of fosfomycin daily in 3 doses and 120–150 mg/kg body weight of oxacillin or cefamandole daily in four doses were administered for 4 to 14 days intravenously (average 10.5 days). After this initial intravenous therapy, treatment was continued orally with clindamycin (25 mg/kg body weight divided into three doses) for a minimum of 3 and a maximum of 8 weeks (mean 4.5 weeks).

Table 2 shows the site of the infectious process and the organisms isolated in the patients in our therapeutic investigation. All organisms were isolated by blood cultures; in antimicrobial sus-

Table 1

Concentrations of fosfomycin in plasma, compact bone and bone marrow
in the rat. Administration of 100 mg/kg body weight IV

	Hours					
	0.5	1	1.5	2	4	6
Plasma	235	132	59	45	8.1	2.6
(µg/ml)	(44)	(30)	(8)	(10)	(5)	(1.1)
Bone marrow	64	42	27	18	2.5	
(µg/g bone)	(19)	(5)	(6)	(4)	(1.7)	
Compact bone	27	26	20	16	7.2	5.0
(µg/g bone)	(6)	(7)	(6)	(9)	(1)	(5.2)

Concentration of fosfomycin in plasma and bone after administration of
75 mg/kg body weight to human volunteers prior to hip replacement

	Concentrations (hours)			
	1	2	3	12
Plasma	284	175	117	17.5
(µg/ml)	(62)	(11)	(36)	(5)
Compact bone	76	44	32	11
(µg/g bone)	(12)	(6)	(8)	(0.1)

ceptibility testing all isolates were susceptible to the antibiotics used
in the clinical trial. In a few patients two or more infectious sites
have been present.

Surgical drainage and decompression was not performed.

The therapeutic outcome of all patients has been reevaluated
within the last 3 months.

Table 2. Bacterial organisms and location of the osteomyelitic focus in patients with acute hematogenous osteomyelitis at the University of Innsbruck, Department of Pediatrics 1980–1986

Staphylocuccus aureus	12	Lower extremity	
H. influenzae	2	Femur	11
Salmonella	1	Tibia	11
Enterobacter	1	Patella	1
Streptococcus pneum.	1	Fibula	2
No organism isolated	13	Calcaneus	3
with previous anti-		Upper extremity	
microbial therapy	9	Humerus	6
		Radius	3
Total	30	Phalanges	4
		Ribs	1
		Clavicle	1
		Mandible	1
		Frontal bone	1
		Sacroiliac joint	1
		Total	46

Results

Results of Experimental Investigations

Fig. 2 shows a photomicrograph of phagocytes with ingested staphylococci. Several staphylococci are seen within phagocytic vacuoles. In contrast to enteric organisms staphylococci lodge in phagocytic vacuoles and are not digested for several hours. The arrow shows a phagosome with a proliferating organism.

Fig. 3 shows kill kinetics of Staphylococcus aureus (MIC $0.5\,\mu g/ml$) in broth with and without granulocytes after addition of cefamandole $50\,\mu g/ml$ in compartment II eluted with a halflife of 1.5 hours. The solid bar shows the number of viable staphylococci within granulocytes after 8 hours. β lactam antibiotics penetrate poorly into phagocytes. This is well demonstrated by the survival of large numbers of staphylococci in granulocytes despite of cefamandole in the broth.

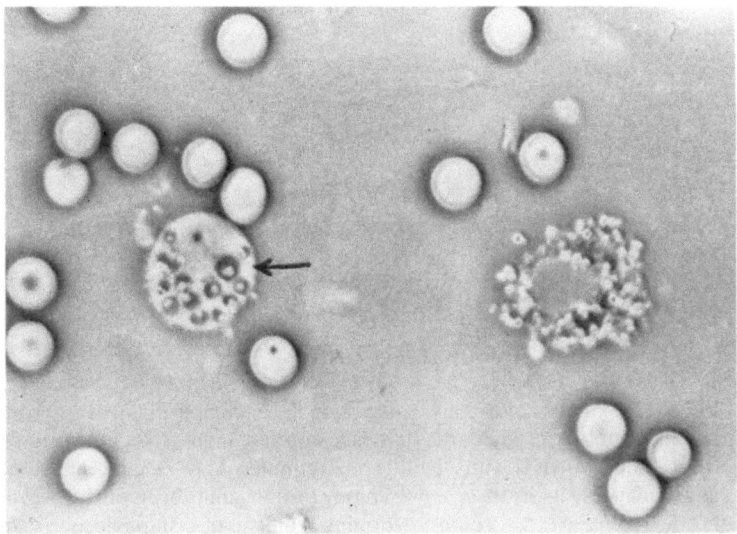

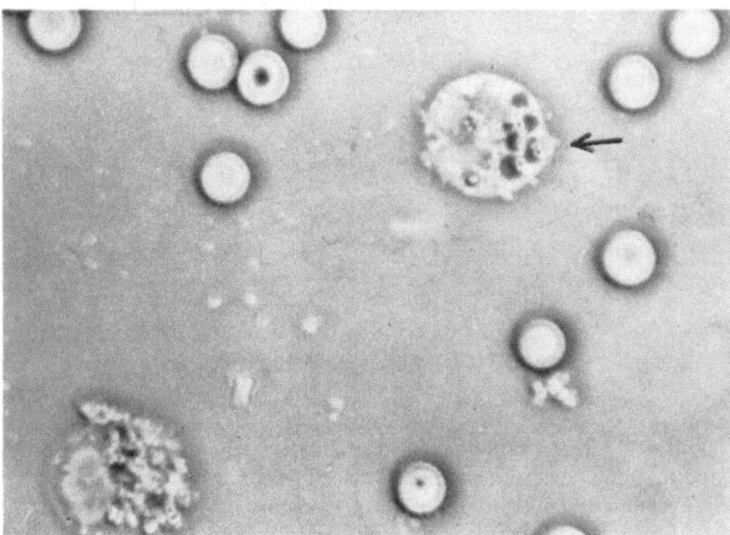

Fig. 2. Phagocytes with intracellular staphylococci 8 hours after administration of cefamandole. The arrow shows proliferating staphylococci within phagocytic vacuoles

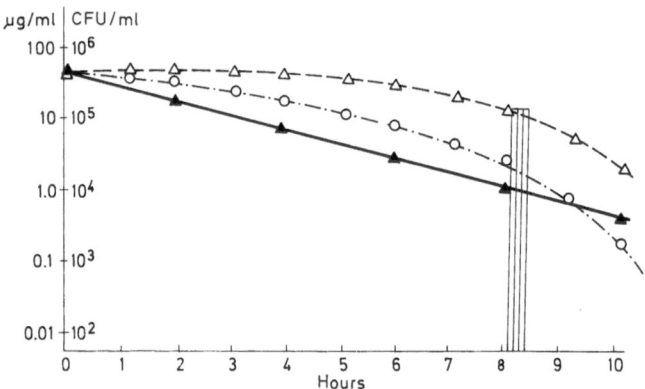

Fig. 3. Kill kinetics of Staphylococcus aureus in compartment II in broth and in granulocytes under the influence of cefamandole (50 μg/ml) eluted from compartment II with a halflife of 90 minutes. ▲——▲ concentrations of cefamandole in broth, △ − − △ colony forming units of staphylococci in broth, ○ − · − · − ○ colony forming units of staphylococci in broth + serum + granulocytes, ▥ colony forming units of staphylococci within 10^6 granulocytes

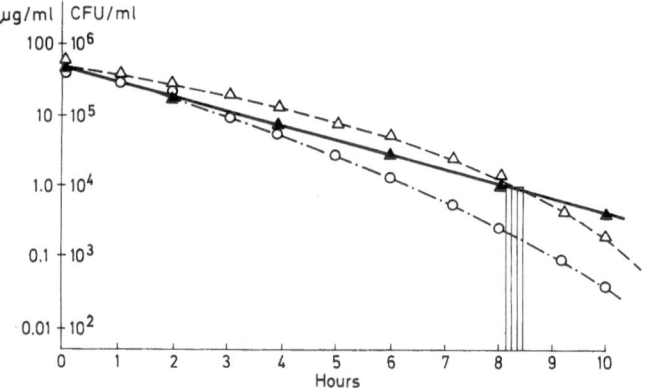

Fig. 4. Kill kinetics of Staphylococcus aureus in compartment II in broth and in granulocytes under the influence of fosfomycin (50 μg/ml) eluted from compartment II with a halflife of 90 minutes. ▲——▲ concentrations of fosfomycin in broth, △ − − △ colony forming unit of staphylococci in broth, ○ − · − · − ○ colony forming units of staphylococci in broth + serum + granulocytes, ▥ colony forming units of staphylococci within 10^6 granulocytes

Other antimicrobial agents like fosfomycin and clindamycin are known to penetrate well into granulocytes and phagocytic vacuoles. This was investigated further in this model.

Fig. 4 shows kill kinetics of Staphylococcus aureus (MIC

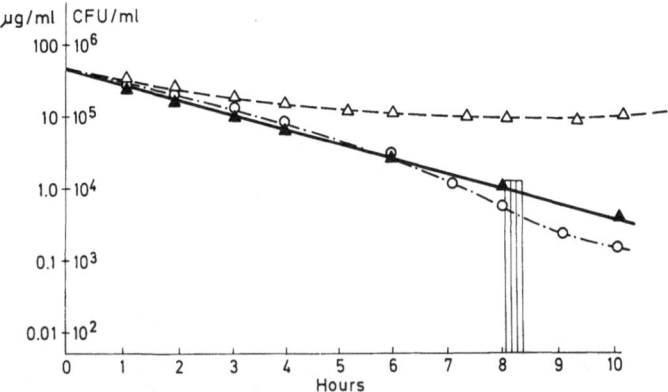

Fig. 5. Kill kinetics of Staphylococcus aureus in compartment II in broth and in granulocytes under the influence of clindamycin (25 µg/ml) eluted from compartment II with a halflife of 90 minutes. ▲——▲ concentrations of clindamycin in broth, △ − − △ colony forming units of staphylococci in broth, ○ −·−·− ○ colony forming units of staphylococci in broth + serum + granulocytes, ⊞ colony forming units of staphylococci within 10^6 granulocytes

0.1 µg/ml) in broth with and without granulocytes under the influence of fluctuating concentrations of fosfomycin 50 µg/ml eliminated from compartment II with a halflife of 1.5 hours. Staphylococci are eliminated considerably faster within the first hours under the influence of fosfomycin than with β lactam antibiotics. The bar shows viable organisms within granulocytes 8 hours after the begin of the experiment.

Fig. 5 shows kill kinetics of Staphylococcus aureus under the influence of fluctuating concentrations of clindamycin (25 µg/ml) in broth alone and with addition of plasma and granulocytes; the solid bar again shows the number of surviving staphylococci within granulocytes.

Both antibiotics, fosfomycin and clindamycin exhibit a much higher reduction in the number of viable organisms within phagocytes than β lactam antibiotics. The numbers of viable organisms are 10 times lower than after addition of cefamandole.

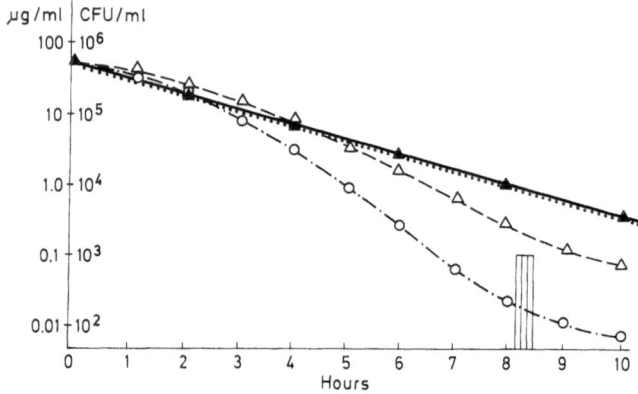

Fig. 6. Kill kinetics of Staphylococcus aureus in compartment II in broth and in granulocytes under the influence of cefamandole (50 µg/ml) in combination with fosfomycin (50 µg/ml) eluted from compartment II with a halflife of 90 minutes. ▲——▲ concentrations of cefamandole in broth, ▲······▲ concentrations of fosfomycin in broth, △ − − △ colony forming units of staphylococci in broth, ○ −·−·− ○ colony forming units of staphylococci in broth + serum + granulocytes, ▥ colony forming units of staphylococci within 10^6 granulocytes

Additional findings in this investigation were:

1. Experiments show a bacteriostatic mode of action of clindamycin on this strain of staphylococcus aureus grown in broth. With the addition of plasma and granulocytes however we observe a bactericidal effect.

2. Bacteria growing under the influence of clindamycin loose their ability to lyse sheep red blood cells within 2 hours as well as their plasma-coagulase activity within 3–4 hours.

Fig. 6 shows kill kinetics of Staphylococcus aureus in broth, in serum plus granulocytes and within granulocytes after adminis-

tration of a combination of cefamandole (50 µg/ml) and fosfomycin (50 µg/ml) eluted with a halflife of 1.5 hours.

Fig. 7 shows kill kinetics of this strain of staphylococcus aureus
under the influence of fosfomycin (50 µg/ml) in combination with

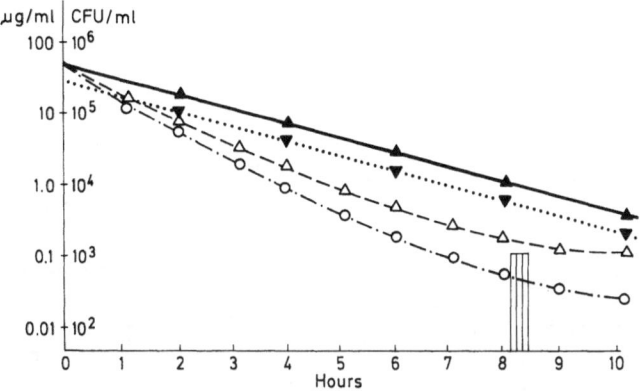

Fig. 7. Kill kinetics of Staphylococcus aureus in compartment II in broth
and in granulocytes under the influence of cefamandole (50 µg/ml) in
combination with clindamycin (25 µg/ml) eluted from compartment II with
a halflife of 90 minutes. ▲——▲ concentrations of cefamandole in broth,
▼······▼ concentrations of clindamycin in broth, △ − − △ colony forming
units of staphylococci in broth, ○ −·−·− ○ colony forming units of
staphylococci in broth + serum + granulocytes, ▥ colony forming units of
staphylococci within 10^6 granulocytes

clindamycin (25 µg/ml) eluted with a halflife of 1.5 hours, in serum
and in granulocytes.

Our data indicate that β lactam antibiotics alone have a limited
effect on bacteria already ingested by macrophages. In contrast,
fosfomycin and clindamycin penetrate favorably into phagocytes
and also kill intracellular ingested staphylococci. Any combination
of these antibiotics shows a synergistic mode of action by reducing
bacteria in broth faster than either drug alone. Also the number of
surviving bacteria in phagocytes was lower by 1–2 log under the
influence of a combination of a β lactam antibiotic and either
fosfomycin or clindamycin.

The combination of clindamycin with fosfomycin showed synergistic activity in broth and granulocytes and was able to eliminate staphylococci from broth and granulocytes almost completely (Fig. 8).

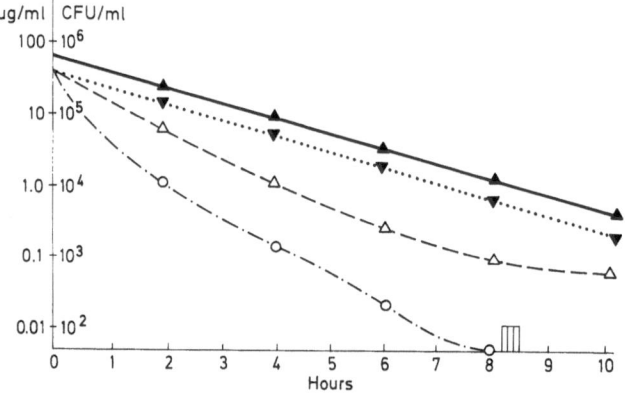

Fig. 8. Kill kinetics of Staphylococcus aureus in compartment II in broth and in granulocytes under the influence of fosfomycin (50 µg/ml) in combination with clindamycin (25 µg/ml) eluted from compartment II with a halflife of 90 minutes. ▲——▲ concentrations of fosfomycin in broth, ▼······▼ concentrations of clindamycin in broth, △ − − △ colony forming units of staphylococci in broth, ○ −·−·− ○ colony forming units of staphylococci in broth + serum + granulocytes, ▥ colony forming units of staphylococci within 10^6 granulocytes

Results of Clinical Investigations

All 30 patients in the study have been treated on a conservative basis with the above-mentioned therapeutic regimen. No surgical procedure was performed. The therapeutic results were excellent. In one patient fosfomycin therapy had to be discontinued due to a questionable bone marrow depression. 29 patients have been treated successfully without sequelae and without functional disturbances. Complete healing of the affected bone was documented radiographically in all patients but one in whom a cosmetic, but not functional defect was seen.

Discussion

Investigations of phagocytosis and its intracellular elimination of a particular strain of Staphylococcus aureus indicate that this isolate from a patient with acute hematogenous osteomyelitis is able to resist intracellular killing for hours. It has been demonstrated in the literature that certain strains of Staphylococcus aureus are able to form an alpha leucocidin, which may block the oxidative burst of granulocytes [7].

These findings allow us to propose an additional pathomechanism for acute hematogenous osteomyelitis in infants and children. Certain strains of Staphylococcus aureus are able to resist intracellular killing and are even able to multiply within a phagocytic vacuole. If one of these strains invades the bloodstream bacteria are rapidly taken up but not destroyed by phagocytes most abundant in the bone marrow. Surviving bacteria within phagocytes may be able to kill the phagocyte, thereby releasing more bacteria. Eventually an abscess formes.

Eradication of these organisms is possible with a combination of a β lactam antibiotic with an antibiotic with intracellular penetration, e.g., fosfomycin or clindamycin. Both antibiotics are highly active against staphylococci, the most frequently isolated organism in this disorder.

This theoretical concept was proven by the successful treatment of 29 patients with acute hematogenous osteomyelitis.

References

1. Adam D (1975) Osteomyelitis im Kindesalter. In: Joppich G, Kienitz M, Marget W, Schönfeld H (Hrsg) Bakterielle Infektionen im Kindesalter. Hahneklee-Symposium, S 174–190
2. Robbins SL Pyogenic osteomyelitis. In: Robbins SL (ed) Pathology. Saunders, Philadelphia London
3. Konzert W, Pillwein K (1981) Die akute hämatogene Osteomyelitis im Kindesalter. Vortrag, Jahrestagung, Österr Gesellschaft für Kinderheilkunde, Bregenz
4. Böyum A (1968) Isolation of mononuclear cells from human blood: isolation of mononuclear cells by one centrifugation and of granulocytes

88   J. P. Guggenbichler et al.: Resistance of Intracellular Killing

by combining centrifugation and sedimentation. Scand J Lab Invest 21 [Suppl] 97: 77–89
5. Guggenbichler JP, König P, Semenitz E, Foisner W (1986) Kill kinetics of bacteria under fluctuating concentrations of various antibiotics II. Chemotherapy 32: 44–52
6. Kerschbaumer F, Guggenbichler JP, Kienel G (1980) Penetration von Fosfomycin in den Knochen im Tierversuch und beim Menschen. Therapiewoche 30: 8173–8177
7. Seeger S (1984) Chronic granulomatous disease: Different treatment modalities. Acta Helv Paed 45: 244–253

Authors' address: Doz. Dr. J. P. Guggenbichler, Universitäts-Kinderklinik, Anichstrasse 35, A-6020 Innsbruck, Austria.

Fosfomycin in the Treatment of Severe Urinary Tract Infections

H. J. Peters

Urologische Klinik, St.-Elisabeth-Krankenhaus, Köln,
Federal Republic of Germany

Summary

70 patients suffering from severe urinary tract infection were treated with 3 × 5 g fosfomycin administered by IV infusion. Fosfomycin concentrations were determined in serum and urine and showed high bactericidal levels. No cumulation was observed in patients with impaired renal function.

The overall clinical success rate in our patients was 91%. 89% of the primary infecting bacteria were eliminated including 8 of 9 strains of Pseudomonas aeruginosa. Relapse was seen in 9%, 6% showed reinfection and 3% a persistent infection.

Patients were particularly observed for the development of side effects. 18 patients were closely scrutinized for renal side effects by serial determinations of creatinine clearance; normal values allow to rule out nephrotoxicity. There was essentially no influence on liver function. Most of the side effects observed were of gastrointestinal nature and could be prevented by a slow infusion rate.

Examination of serum electrolytes in 20 patients with normal renal function and balance studies in 6 further patients showed no signs of hypernatremia inspite of a supply of 218 mmol sodium given with 15 g of fosfomycin. The excretion of sodium and potassium in the urine was greatly enhanced. Occasionally the development of hypokalemia was seen on the 2nd and 3rd day. Potassium substitution is recommended therefore in the case of low initial serum potassium concentrations. Electrolytes in 10 patients showed no significant changes if potassium was substituted simultaneously.

Zusammenfassung

70 Patienten mit schweren, meist komplizierten Harnweginfekten wurden mit 3 × 5 g Fosfomycin intravenös als Kurzinfusion behandelt. Die Patienten litten an verschiedenen Grundkrankheiten; Obstruktionen der ableitenden Harnwege wurden bei 48 Patienten vor Behandlung mit Fosfomycin behoben.

Die Empfindlichkeit auf Fosfomycin wurde von 394 klinischen Isolaten von Patienten mit Harnweginfekten geprüft. 89.6% (353 Keime) waren auf Fosfomycin empfindlich, im Vergleich mit β-Laktam-Antibiotika und Aminoglykosiden eine bemerkenswert hohe Empfindlichkeit.

Serum und Harnkonzentrationen wurden bei 11 Patienten mit normaler und 7 Patienten mit eingeschränkter Nierenfunktion in zweitägigen Abständen bestimmt. Auch bei Patienten mit eingeschränkter Nierenfunktion wurde keine Kumulation gefunden. Im Harn werden 45—54% der verabreichten Antibiotikamenge innerhalb von 3 Stunden in aktiver Form ausgeschieden. Harnkonzentrationen sind daher sehr hoch und liegen im Bereich von 4,000 µg/ml.

Die klinische Heilungsrate bei Gabe von 15 g Fosfomycin täglich betrug 90%. Die bakteriologische Beurteilung ergab, daß 89% der Primärisolate — darunter 7 von 8 Pseudomonasisolaten — erfolgreich eliminiert werden konnten. In 9 % der Fälle kam es zum Rezidiv, in 6 % zur Reinfektion, 3% zeigten eine persistierende Infektion.

Besonderes Augenmerk wurde auf die Entwicklung von Nebenwirkungen gelegt. Gastrointestinale Nebenwirkungen mit Nausea und Erbrechen wurden am häufigsten (27%) beobachtet, konnten jedoch mit einer langsameren Infusionsgeschwindigkeit vermieden werden. Andere Nebenwirkungen, insbesondere renale Nebenwirkungen, waren vernachlässigbar gering. Bei 8 Patienten mit eingeschränkter Nierenfunktion wurde die glomeruläre Filtration während der Behandlung mit Fosfomycin verfolgt und sogar eine Besserung beobachtet.

Es erhob sich die Frage, ob 218 mmol Natrium, die mit 15 g Fosfomycin verabreicht werden, zu einer Änderung der Serumelektrolyte führen. Bei keinem der Patienten konnte eine Änderung des Serum-Natrium-Spiegels gefunden werden. Bisweilen, insbesondere wenn zu Behandlungsbeginn bereits niedrige Kaliumwerte im Serum bestanden, kommt es jedoch zur Entwicklung einer Hypokaliämie. Bilanzuntersuchungen zeigten, daß ab dem 3. Behandlungstag die Natriumausscheidung im Harn deutlich ansteigt. Die Kaliumbilanz ist hingegen bereits am ersten Behandlungstag negativ. Substitution mit 60 mmol Kalium in 1—2 l isotoner Infusionslösung wird daher beim Erwachsenen mit initial niedrigem Kaliumspiegel empfohlen. Unter dieser Substitution wurden keine Elektrolytveränderungen beobachtet.

Introduction

Fosfomycin is an interesting new antibiotic with a bactericidal mechanisms of action and a broad range of susceptibility against nosocomial pathogens. Its favorable pharmacokinetic profile such as low protein binding and pk_A value, long halflife of elimination and small molecular size allow for high concentrations in interstitial and extracellular fluids. Fosfomycin is eliminated in the urine in a non-metabolized form. The 24-hours-recovery rate is 98% resulting in very high bactericidal concentrations in urine [1, 2, 3]. Due to its exclusive renal elimination no impact on the fecal flora and emergence of resistent organisms in the fecal flora is expected. It seemed warranted therefore to investigate fosfomycin in the treatment of severe, complicated urinary tract infections.

Clinical Investigation

Material and Methods

In the years 1979 to 1981 an open clinical study to investigate the efficacy and tolerance of fosfomycin was performed in 70 patients with urinary tract infections. Patients suffering from various underlying diseases were treated with 3×5 g of fosfomycin daily. Most patients suffered from chronic recurrent pyelonephritis. Patients with indwelling catheters, acute lower urinary tract infections and asymptomatic bacteriuria were excluded.

Table 1 summarizes data of these patients.

62 patients suffered from complicated urinary tract infection. In 48 cases the obstruction of the urinary tract was removed just before initiation of fosfomycin therapy. Surgery was carried out in 7 patients with simultaneous antibiotic treatment. Further 7 patients had nonremovable obstructions. 8 patients had noncomplicated urinary tract infections. Criteria for enrollment in the study were significant bacteriuria and sensitivity of the infecting organisms to fosfomycin.

For susceptibility testing the disk-test method of Kirby-Bauer on Müller-Hinton agar was used. Discs were loaded with 50 µg

Table 1. Clinical study 1979–1981. Data of patients, localisation of the urinary tract infections (n = 70)

sex		age (median age) in years
men	44	15–81 (62)
women	26	19–74 (40)
Total	70	

	men	women
Obstructive chronic recurrent pyelonephritis	11	17
Obstructive acute pyelonephritis	10	15
Infections of the lower urinary tract with obstructions	2	7
Non complicated UTI	3	5
Total	26	44

Table 2. Sensitivity of 394 organisms isolated from infected urines against fosfomycin from July 1979 to February 1981. (Disc test, Bauer 1966, Mueller-Hinton agar.)

Species	No. of isolates	No. of strains sensitive (moderate sensitive)	resistant
Escherichia coli	247	235 (12)	12
Proteus mirabilis	46	29 (11)	17
Proteus vulgaris	4	2 (1)	2
Pseudomonas aeruginosa	35	29 (9)	6
Klebsiella pneumoniae	25	25 (8)	–
Enterobacter agglomerans	26	23 (9)	3
Enterobacter aerogenes	6	6 (3)	–
Serratia marcescens	5	4 (–)	1
Total	394	353 (53)	41

Table 3. Spectrum of infecting bacteria in 69 patients before and after therapy with fosfomycin

Species	No of strains before therapy	Elimination	Persistance	Relapse	Reinfection
E. coli	47	43*	1	3	1
Pseudomonas aeruginosa	9	8	–	1	–
Proteus mirabilis	5	4	–	1(r)	–
Proteus vulgaris/rettgeri	–	–	–	–	2
Klebsiella pneumoniae	4	3	–	1	1
Enterobacter cloacae/agglomerans	4	4	–	–	–
Serratia marcescens	2	1	1(r)	–	–
Staphylococcus aureus	2	2	–	–	–
Total	73	65	2	6	4
Patients	69	61	2	6	4
mixed infections	4	–	–	–	–

* 1 strain was eliminated by therapy with gentamicin
(r = resistant)

fosfomycin plus 50 µg glucose-6-phosphate. From July 1979 to February 1981 394 gramnegative organisms were isolated from infected urines. Table 2 shows the susceptibility pattern of these 394 organisms. In comparison with β lactam antibiotics and aminglycosides this antibiotic was highly effective against various strains of E. coli, Klebsiella, and Enterobacter.

Results

Clinical and Bacteriological Investigation

Evaluation of the clinical efficacy was possible in only 54 patients. Assessment was based on temperature, leucocytosis, ESR, and a patient questionnaire. Clinical results were satisfactory in 90%. Treatment failure occurred in 10%. Leucocyturia subsided in 73% of patients although most patients underwent surgery before or during therapy. Consequently leucocyturia can not be regarded as good criterion for evaluation.

Table 3 demonstrates bacteriological results 4 days after the end of therapy. 73 bacterial organisms were isolated from 69 patients; 65 strains (89%) were eliminated. In one patient treatment was discontinued due to severe side effects. In 83% of the 69 patients the urine was sterile 4 days after the end of therapy, 9% (6 patients) showed a relapse, 6% (4 patients) developed reinfection and 3% (2 patients) had persistent infection.

Pharmacokinetic Investigation

Serum and urine concentrations of fosfomycin were determined in 11 patients with normal and 7 patients with impaired renal function. Blood samples were taken at the end of fosfomycin infusion on the 2nd, 4th, 6th, and 8th day. Serum concentrations are shown in Table 5. No accumulation of fosfomycin in serum was observed even not in patients with impaired renal function.

Peak concentrations in urine were more than 4,000 mg/l. In the first 3 hours between 45 and 54% of the administered amount of drug was excreted in a microbiologically active form in the urine. Elimination was lower in patients with impaired renal function but concentrations always exceeded substantially the MIC values of all organisms.

Tolerance

Back in 1979 there was little information on the tolerance of the daily dose of 15 g fosfomycin. All patients were therefore thoroughly monitored. The most frequent side effect was nausea affecting 19 of 70 patients. However, infusion time of an hour or more significantly reduced the occurrence of this symptom. Symptoms such as headache and retrosternal pain was reported less frequently. In Table 4 clinical and laboratory side effects are summarized.

In all 70 patients no significant change in serum creatinine concentration occurred ruling out nephrotoxicity. Glomerular filtration rate even increased in 8 patients with impaired renal function while under treatment with fosfomycin.

Further studies concerned possible changes in serum electrolytes. 15 g of fosfomycin is infused with 218 mmol of sodium so that hypertonic hyperhydration may be a threat. At the end of the

Table 4. Side effects in 70 patients treated with fosfomycin (3 × 5 g daily)

side effects	noticed in ... patients
gastrointestinal disorders (nausea, sickness, vomiting, diarrhoea)	19
headache	7
cardialgia	2
outbreak of sweat feeling of weakness	2
genital mycosis	1
thrompophlebitis	1
elevation of transaminase	10
elevation of LAP	10
decrease in the number of leucocytes	3

Table 5. Serum concentrations of fosfomycin in 11 patients with normal renal function and 7 patients with compensated renal insufficiency in μg/ml

	2. day	4. day	6. day	8. day
Patient with normal renal function	374 ± 152	300 ± 133	350 ± 155	323 ± 91
Patients with compensated renal function	345 ± 109	323 ± 124	347 ± 124	423 ± 29

infusion sodium and potassium concentrations were measured in the serum of 12 patients. The mean values were within the normal range, although there was a moderate decrease in potassium concentrations (Table 6). In 8 patients with impaired renal function there was no change in sodium concentration, but a significant decrease in serum potassium. In a further study the electrolyte

Table 6. Mean values of sodium and potassium at the end of the fosfomycin infusion in 12 patients. Serum electrolytes in patients with normal renal function

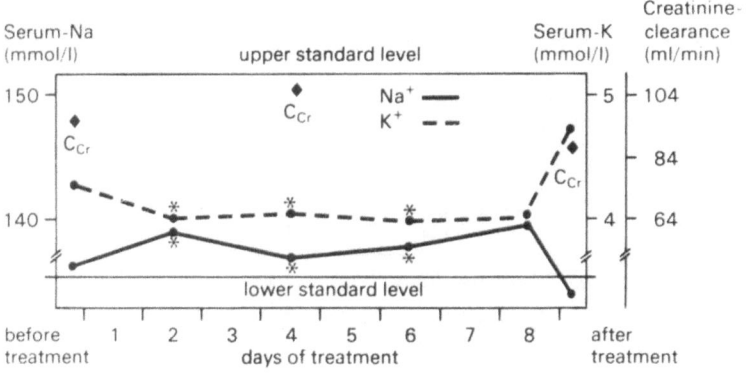

*significant difference (Wilcoxon-Test)

Table 7. Mean values of 6 patients with urospesis. Serum Na$^+$ and serum K$^+$ and balance in patients treated with fosfomycin

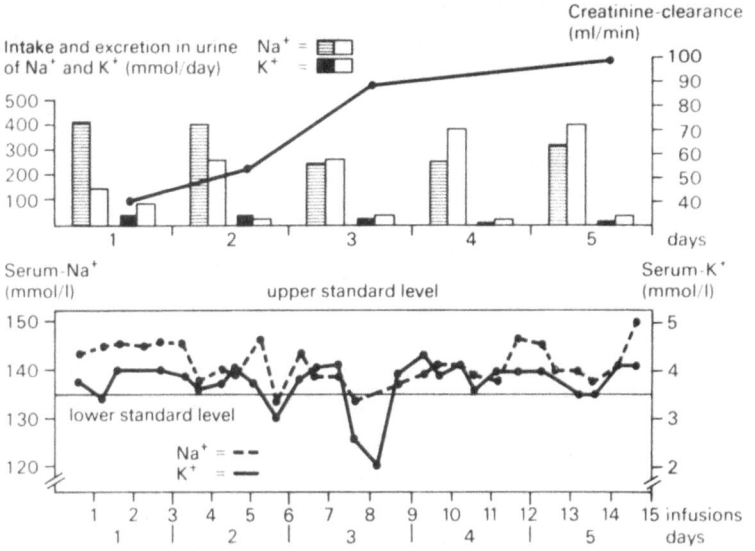

Table 8. Therapy with 15 g fosfomycin and 60 mmol potassium chloride. Excretion of Na^+ and K^+ by 24-hour urine in 10 patients

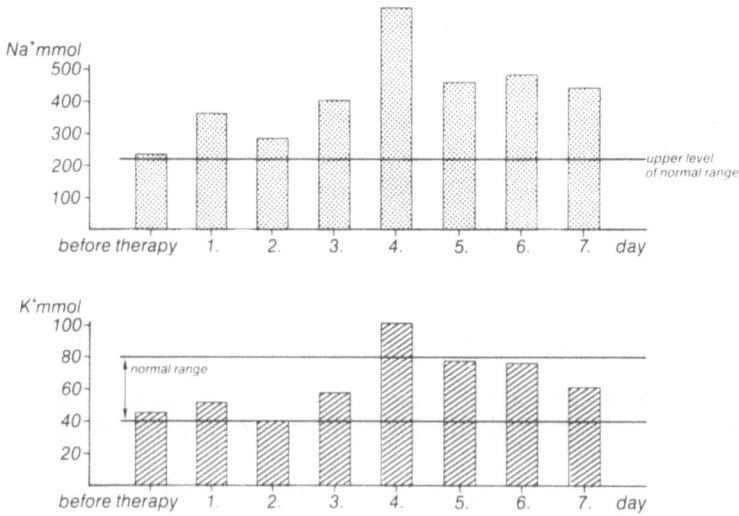

balance was determined in 6 patients with septicemia. Sodium, potassium, chloride, and calcium concentrations were measured in serum 4 times daily as well as intake and excretion of these electrolytes in urine (Table 7). Initially sodium concentrations were low and intake was higher than excretion. As of the third day the excretion of sodium exceeded the intake rate and occasional hyponatremia was observed. There was a negative potassium balance from the first day resulting in hypokalemia already on the second day of treatment, in some cases serious enough to require compensation. Therefore since hypokalemia may develop after 2–3 days (especially if potassium concentrations were low to begin with) 15 g of fosfomycin was combined with 60 mmol of potassium chloride in 2–3 liters of isotonic solutions in 10 patients. In this prospective study serum electrolytes remained normal. Table 8 demonstrates the excessively high sodium excretion and the analogue increase of potassium excretion during this treatment.

Conclusion

Our study recommends fosfomycin for the treatment of severe complicated urinary tract invection. Fosfomycin is well tolerated if infusion time takes at least one hour. No signs of nephrotoxicity were found. Disturbances in electrolytes can be avoided by the administration of 60 mmol potassium chloride in isotonic solutions.

References

1. Guggenbichler JP, Kienel G, Frisch H (1978) Fosfomycin, ein neues Antibiotikum. Pharmakokinetische Untersuchungen bei Kindern, Früh- und Neugeborenen. Pädiatr Pädol 13: 429–436
2. Kawabata N, Shiraha J, et al (1978) A study on serum level and urinary excretion of fosfomycin-Na in man with special reference to pharmacokinetic analysis. Jpn J Antibiot 31: 549–560
3. Kolb R, Kienel G (1979) Comparison of the kinetics of fosfomycin in plasma and wound exudates. Proct 10th int congr chemother, Zürich, pp 682–683

Author's address: Dr. H. J. Peters, Urologische Klinik, St.-Elisabeth-Krankenhaus, D-5000 Köln-Hohenlind, Federal Republic of Germany.

Penetration of Fosfomycin into Heart Valves, Subcutaneous and Muscle Tissue of Patients Undergoing Open Heart Surgery

R. Achatzy, F. Daschner, N. Pittlik, und F. Bartels

Chirurgische Klinik und Poliklinik, Universität Münster,
Federal Republic of Germany

Summary

54 adult patients undergoing open heart surgery were given a 5 g fosfomycin infusion preoperatively. Pharmacokinetics and tissue penetration of fosfomycin was determined. Peak concentrations of fosfomycin were reached within the heart (valve, muscle and subcutaneous tissue) after 30–60 minutes. In many cases they exceeded the corresponding serum concentrations. No difference in serum elimination of fosfomycin was noticed during cardiac bypass compared with normal patients.

Fosfomycin concentrations in heart valves exceeded MIC values of most grampositive and gramnegative organisms causing postoperative wound infections and endocarditis.

No side effects were observed.

Zusammenfassung

Staphylokokkus aureus und Staphylokokkus epidermidis werden häufig, E. coli und Klebsiella pneumoniae seltener als Erreger von Wundinfektionen und Endokarditis nach Herzoperationen isoliert. Wesentliche Aspekte einer erfolgreichen antimikrobiellen Chemotherapie sind einerseits eine hohe Empfindlichkeit gegen die am häufigsten isolierten Keime, anderseits die Penetration in (einen) den Infektionsherd. Bisher verfügbare Antibiotika zeigen ein hohes Maß an Resistenz gegen diese multipel resistenten Hospitalkeime, zudem penetrieren sie ungenügend ins bradytrophe Gewebe von z. B.

narbig veränderten Herzklappen. Außerdem wird die Pharmakokinetik verschiedener Antibiotika durch den kardiopulmonalen Bypass verändert.

In dieser Untersuchung wurde daher die Penetration von Fosfomycin nach Gabe von 5 g der Substanz in Form einer intravenösen Kurzinfusion präoperativ in Serum, ins Myokard, in Herzklappen, ins subkutane Gewebe und in Muskelgewebe untersucht.

54 Patienten, 14 davon mit Koronargefäßrekonstruktion, 40 mit Klappenersatzoperationen, wurden in die Untersuchung einbezogen.

Die Untersuchungen zeigen, daß die Maximalkonzentration von Fosfomycin im Herzen (Klappengewebe, Muskulatur, subkutanes Fettgewebe) bereits nach 30—60 Minuten erreicht wird. In vielen Fällen übertreffen die Gewebekonzentrationen die korrespondierenden Serumkonzentrationen. Insbesondere im Myokard werden hohe Konzentrationen gefunden. Es scheint, daß Antibiotika, insbesondere Fosfomycin, von der Plasmaseite und nicht vom Interstitium ins Klappengewebe diffundieren. Ein kardiopulmonaler Bypaß hat keinen Einfluß auf die Kinetik und Gewebepenetration von Fosfomycin.

Mit den betreffenden Gewebekonzentrationen werden 99% Staphylococcus aureus, 98% von E. coli und 68% von Klebsiella pneumoniae gehemmt.

Diese Daten zeigen, daß Fosfomycin sowohl in der Prophylaxe als auch in der Behandlung von postoperativen Infektionen des Herzens empfohlen werden kann.

Introduction

In postoperative wound infections and late endocarditis following open heart surgery multiple resistant nosocomial organisms are isolated. Another important aspect for effective antibacterial therapy is an appropriate concentration of the antibiotic at the site of the suspected infection. Most available antibiotics are either insensitive to these difficult to treat organisms and/or diffuse poorly into the bradytrophic tissue of scarred heart valves. In addition pharmacokinetics of various antibiotics, e.g. β lactam antibiotics are frequently altered by cardiopulmonary bypass.

In the present study the distribution of fosfomycin—an antibiotic with a broad spectrum of activity in serum, muscle, subcutaneous tissue, bone and especially in scarred heart valves—was investigated in patients undergoing open heart surgery most of them with cardiopulmonary bypass.

Material and Methods

Patient Profile

During the study lasting from January to November 1984 14 patients with coronary heart disease (12 men, 2 women) with a mean age of 56.9 years and a mean weight of 70.3 kg were operated. All these patients suffered from severe coronary artery sclerosis, generally with multiple coronary vessel disease; an average of 2.3 coronary vessels were revascularized with autologous veins.

In the same period 40 patients, 28 men, 12 women with a mean age of 56 years, mean weight of 62.4 kg, underwent surgery for acquired cardiac valve defects.

15 of these patients received prosthetic aortic valve replacement,

13 prosthetic mitral valve replacement,

4 prosthetic aortic and mitral valve replacement,

2 patients underwent open mitral valve commisurotomy,

5 patients had prosthetic aortic valve replacement with coronary reconstruction and

1 patient received prosthetic mitral valve replacement with coronary reconstruction.

All patients had normal renal function and received 5 g of fosfomycin preoperatively by infusion over 30 minutes.

Operation Technique

After median sternotomy and periocardiotomy the ascending aorta, both venae cavae and occasionally the right atrium were cannulized and the patients were attached to the heart lung machine. After transition to total cardiopulmonary bypass and transverse clamping of the ascending aorta operation was performed under moderate hypothermia and in cardioplegic arrest with "Bretschneiders solution" applied by the aortic route. The pump was primed with 1,000 ml Ringer's lactate solution, 500 ml of whole blood, 200 ml of osmofundin (Braun Melsungen) and 40 ml of trisbuffer. Nonpulsatile blood flow was maintained at 50 ml/kg/min during cardiac bypass and blood temperature was kept at 25–35 °C. The mean arterial pressure varied from 60–80 mm Hg. The mean extra-corporal circulation time was 90 minutes.

As valve prosthesis a tilting plate prosthesis of the typ "omni-science" was implanted.

After rewarming, the patient was resuscitated and the heart decannulated after removal of the extracorporal bypass. After applying protamine effecting hemostasis and inserting two substernal drains, the thorax was closed again in layers.

Samples and Antibiotic Assays

Blood was taken simultaneously at various intervals following infusion of fosfomycin from the venous line, subcutaneous fat and muscle. Tissue samples and blood were taken at the time of valve replacement. Adherent blood was removed from the tissue specimen by sterile gauze. The specimen were immediately frozen at — 72 °C and assayed during the following week by an agar diffusion method using E. coli 106 as test organism (spore suspension: BBL; antibiotic medium number 2, Oxoid).

Tissue fluid was obtained in tris-HCl-buffer dilution (pH 7.2) by means of a Coleworth stomacher number 80.

Standards for plasma and antibiotic assays were made in Tris-HCl-buffered human serum (1 : 1), for tissue fluid in buffer pH 7.2. All analyses were performed in triplicate. Some tissue samples, however, were too small for determination of concentration.

Results

Table 1 shows concentrations of antibiotics in serum and tissue from patients with coronary heart disease at various times. Within 180 minutes mean serum concentrations decreased from 196 to 138 µg/ml. Average fosfomycin concentrations in subcutaneous and muscle tissue were between 98 µg/g and 32.5 µg/g. Results of fosfomycin concentrations in fat and muscle tissue should be interpreted with great caution because of the small number of cases.

Table 1. Plasma and tissue concentrations after infusion of 5 g fosfomycin (µg/ml; g). Patients with coronary heart disease

	0–60 minutes	60–120 minutes	120–180 minutes
Plasma	195,74 SD ± 82,30 (23)	128,6 SD ± 41.61 (35)	138 SD ± 12.31 (6)
Myocardial and subcutaneous tissue	98 SD ± 52.49 (7)	26 (1)	32.5 (2)

Number of patients: 14; mean weight: 78.1 kg; mean age: 56.9 years.

Table 2. Plasma and tissue concentrations after infusion of 5 g fosfomycin (µg/ml; g): Patients with cardiac valve defects

	0–60 minutes	60–120 minutes	120–180 minutes
Plasma	156,13 SD ± 61.56 (31)	132.12 SD ± 36.48 (26)	—
Heart valve	87.52 SD ± 56.00 (21)	80.1 SD ± 51.70 (10)	—
Myocardial tissue	178 (2)	95.62 SD ± 60.15 (16)	92.43 SD ± 51.49 (7)

Number of patients: 40; mean weight: 62.4 kg; mean age: 56 years.

Table 2 shows concentrations of antibiotics in serum and tissue from patients with acquired cardiac valve defects at various times. The serum concentrations varied between 156 µg/ml and 132 µg/ml within 120 minutes.

In heart valves the concentration decreased from 87.5 µg/g to

80 µg/g. The highest concentrations were found in myocardial tissue. They decreased from 178 µg/g in the first hour to 92 µg/g in the third hour.

Discussion

Staphylococcus aureus and Staphylococcus epidermidis are isolated as the most frequent pathogens of postoperative wound infections and late endocarditis following open heart surgery. Gramnegative organisms like E. coli and Klebsiella pneumoniae can be isolated from the blood and prosthetic heart valves of patients with early onset postoperative endocarditis. Fosfomycin concentration in heart valves are high enough to inhibit most of these pathogens. 99% of Staphylococcus aureus, 97% of E. coli and 68% of Klebsiella are inhibited at a fosfomycin concentration of 16 µg/ml. Actual fosfomycin concentrations in myocardial tissue, in heart valves and subcutaneous tissue are substantially higher.

Antibiotics and expecially fosfomycin seem to diffuse into the heart valves from the plasma rather than from the interstitial space. The serum concentrations in patients undergoing open heart surgery correlate well with those in healthy volunteers. In contrast to other antibiotics such as cephalosporins, the pharmacokinetics of fosfomycin do not seem to be significantly influenced by cardiopulmonary bypass.

No side effects due to fosfomycin were registered.

Conclusion

Since fosfomycin penetrates tissue well, diffuses even into brady-throphic tissue of scarred heart valves and most organisms are sensitive to it, this new antimicrobial substance can be recommended for prophylaxis and treatment of cardiovascular infections.

Authors' address: Prof. Dr. R. Achatzy, Thorax- und Gefäßchirurgie, Speziallungenklinik Hemer, Postfach 360/380, D-5870 Hemer, Federal Republic of Germany.

Fosfomycin in the Treatment of Pulmonary Infections Combined with Heart Failure

C. Krüger

Innere Abteilung, Krankenhaus Alten Eichen, Hamburg,
Federal Republic of Germany

Summary

32 patients with bronchopulmonary infections were treated with fosfomycin in various doses. Therapeutic success was verified in 30 patients. Particular attention was paid to recording adverse reactions on the heart and circulation. Parameters used were the central venous pressure and the right ventricular diameter measured sonographically. These parameters increased in 3 of 7 patients suffering from heart failure based on coronary heart disease or toxic myocarditis. Two of these patients showed signs of congestive right heart failure normalizing after discontinuation of fosfomycin therapy. In two further patients a slightly increased central venous pressure was recorded without clinical symptoms.

It follows that in patients with decompensated congestive heart failure fosfomycin therapy should be discontinued and continuous monitoring of the central venous pressure is recommended thereafter.

If the organisms causing subacute or chronic bacterial infections with possible prior tissue damage or abscess formation are sensitive to fosfomycin, this antibiotic is indicated. The favorable pharmacokinetic properties of fosfomycin with high serum and tissue concentrations justify its use.

Zusammenfassung

32 Patienten mit bronchopulmonalen Infektionen wurden mit 2 bzw. 3 × 5 g Fosfomycin intravenös in Form einer Kurzinfusion behandelt. Der Großteil dieser Patienten wurde bereits zuvor mit verschiedenen Cephalospori-

nen bzw. Aminoglykosiden erfolglos behandelt. Ein therapeutischer Erfolg wurde bei 30 Patienten beobachtet.

Besonderes Augenmerk wurde auf die Registrierung von Nebenwirkungen auf Herz und Kreislauf gelegt. Als Parameter dienten der zentrale Venendruck und der echokardiographisch gemessene rechtsventrikuläre Herzdurchmesser. Von 7 Patienten mit rekompensierter Herzinsuffizienz auf dem Boden einer koronaren Herzerkrankung bzw. einer toxischen Myokarditis reagierten 3 mit Anstieg der genannten Parameter. Der zentrale Venendruck war bei 2 Patienten auf das Doppelte des Normalwertes erhöht. Diese 2 Patienten entwickelten auch eine diskrete klinische Symptomatik. 2 Patienten zeigten einen leicht erhöhten zentralen Venendruck ohne klinische Symptomatik. Daraus wird gefolgert, daß Patienten mit Herzinsuffizienz von einer Behandlung mit Fosfomycin ausgenommen werden sollten, und daß nach Rekompensation eine engmaschige Kontrolle z. B. des zentralen Venendrucks anzuraten ist.

Unter der Voraussetzung einer günstigen In-vitro-Sensibilität sehen wir die Indikation von Fosfomycin bei akut bis chronisch verlaufenden bakteriellen Infektionen mit Gewebeschädigung bzw. Abszedierung, die erfolglos vorbehandelt wurden. Dann steht in Fosfomycin ein hochwirksames Präparat zur Verfügung. Die günstigen pharmakokinetischen Eigenheiten dieser Substanz mit hohen Serum- und Gewebekonzentrationen sind wahrscheinlich für die klinischen Erfolge mitverantwortlich.

Introduction

Fosfomycin is an antibiotic embracing a broad spectrum of clinically relevant grampositive and gramnegative pathogens [1]. Moreover, the penetrating capabilities of this small molecule are responsible for the high serum and tissue concentrations observed in previous investigations [2].

Reservations concerning the use of this antibiotic for pulmonary infections had been mentioned because of the risk of potential cardiovascular stress as a result of the high sodium content.

Particular attention has been paid to these adverse reactions by means of a clinical study concerning the efficacy of fosfomycin in bronchopulmonary bacterial infections.

Material and Methods

5 g of fosfomycin BID oder TID were administered parenterally over 5 days to 32 patients with bacterial bronchopulmonary

infections. A large number of these patients had been previously treated with various antibacterial substances without success. An orotracheobronchial organism count was carried out in 22 patients using the Krüger method [3]. Blood cultures were performed regularly. Therapeutic success was recorded clinically and radiographically.

In order to observe right ventricular strain, we recorded the central venous pressure and the diameter of the right ventricle sonographically before and after fosfomycin (5 g) over 5 days in a total of 5 patients. Central venous pressure alone was recorded in 2 additional patients. Electrocardiograms and daily electrolyte checks were also carried out.

6 of these 7 patients were already suffering from congestive heart failure, one patient had a toxic myocarditis. All patients were compensated at the beginning of therapy in spite of the right ventricular strain due to the underlying pulmonary pathology.

Results

The most dominant organism detected was Streptococcus pneumoniae (6 ×) followed by Klebsiella pneumoniae (3 ×) and Streptococcus pyogenes (2 ×). E. coli, H. influenzae and Staphylococcus aureus were isolated once. Pathogens with questionable clinical relevance were Neisseria spp., Serratia marcescens and Staphylococcus epidermidis. No organism could be isolated either by blood culture or by tracheobronchial aspiration in the remaining 15 cases. Of 17 isolated organisms only 2 were insensitive to fosfomycin.

A favorable therapeutic effect was observed in 30 patients despite prior unsuccessful therapy using antibiotics in accordance with the antibiogram. Of the two nonresponsive patients one exhibited a fosfomycin resistant organism. This patient with a Klebsiella pneumoniae infection and cardiac congestion was not improved by fosfomycin therapy. In another patient with chronic bronchitis and dilatation of the bronchi a transient effect was observed: germ mutation occurred. Although a fosfomycin susceptible klebsiella had been cultured initially, proteus mirabilis was isolated at the end of therapy. In addition a relaps of right basal pneumonia occurred as a result of heart failure of unclear etiology after there had been a definite improvement initially.

The following is a report of a 82-year-old patient with exsudative left basal pleuropneumonia and heart failure. Initial therapy with a cephalosporin and aminoglycoside combination administered over 6 days remained unsuccessful. After switching to 5 g fosfomycin BID the patient was afebrile on the second day of treatment. After 5 days fosfomycin was discontinued. However, fever returned so that therapy was reassumed for 9 more days. By this time the patient was well again.

Particular attention was paid to adverse reactions of fosfomycin therapy: Although no disturbances in electrolyte metabolism were found a clear right ventricular strain was verified in 3 of 7 patients with several parameters. The right ventricular diameter of one patient with normal central venous pressure increased significantly after 5 g of fosfomycin therapy TID over 5 days. The patient was well clinically, all values normalized again after discontinuing therapy. The other two patients showed an increase in central venous pressure to more than 20 mm H_2O after 5 g fosfomycin BID over 6 days and developed signs of clear pulmonary congestion. These findings also normalized after discontinuation of therapy. Finally we recorded a slight increase in the central venous pressure in two other patients without clinical symptoms. It also should be noted, that two of the former patients showed congestion induced moderate renal failure.

Discussion

The clinical efficacy of fosfomycin to bacterial bronchopneumonia is convincing if the organisms is sensitive to fosfomycin. 28 patients showed a excellent clinical response, two a moderate response to fosfomycin. In two patients therapeutic failure was noted. Similar good results could be shown in earlier studies. Once again we were able to establish a particularly favorable action of fosfomycin in vivo possibly as a result of its good pharmacokinetic properties. The use of fosfomycin should be considered where other therapy has proven ineffective with subacute to chronic courses of infection in previously damaged tissue or where abscesses have formed. The adverse reaction of this substance on the cardiovascular system however should be taken into consideration because of its relatively high sodium content and therefore osmotic activity. Although this affects only a few cases, fosfomycin should not be used when heart damage or congestive failure is present due to the sodium loading and consequent hypervolemia.

References

1. Grimm H (1979) In vitro investigations with fosfomycin on Mueller-Hinten Agar with an without glucose-6-phosphate. Infection 7: 256–259
2. Sicilia T, Estevez E, Rodriguez A (1981) Fosfomycin penetration into the cerebrospinal fluid of patients with bacterial meningitis. Chemotherapy 27: 405–413
3. Krüger Ch (1983) Orotracheobronchiale Aspiration zur bakteriologischen und cytologischen Diagnostik. Dtsch Med Wochenschr 108: 1395–1399

Author's address: Prof. Dr. C. Krüger, Innere Abteilung, Krankenhaus Alten Eichen, Jütländer Allee 48, D-2000 Hamburg, Federal Republic of Germany.

Fosfomycin in Cystic Fibrosis

H. Meyer

Alpine Kinderklinik Pro Juventute, Davos, Switzerland

Summary

In a series of 86 patients (49 females, 37 males) suffering from cystic fibrosis fosfomycin has been administered in a therapeutic investigation in duration of 1–4 weeks. Patients varied between 4 and 37 years. All patients have received previous antimicrobial therapy for years with little improvement. The pulmonary condition of our patients varied from moderately to severely damaged lungs. In the majority of patients various strains of Pseudomonas aeruginosa in combination with other pathogenic and facultative pathogenic bacteria were isolated. Routine susceptibility testing showed a high degree (90%) of resistance to fosfomycin. Problems with antimicrobial susceptibility testing were encountered: organisms found resistant in disc diffusion tests exhibited sensitivity well within the therapeutic range by a tube dilution test. Favorable clinical results of a pilot study showed improvement in the general condition of the patients despite of resistance in routine in vitro testing: These facts encouraged us to proceed with the clinical investigation of fosfomycin.

Fosfomycin was administered once daily in a 30–40 minutes intravenous infusion. The dosage was adapted to body weight. The duration of treatment varied according to the severity of the condition.

Fosfomycin was well tolerated; no hematological, renal, hepatic, allergic, neurologic or circulatory side effects were noted. Although an overall assessment of the therapeutic results was difficult because numerous conditions unrelated to antimicrobial therapy like nutrition, optimal physicotherapy etc. are influencing the disease and various combinations with other antibiotics were used, we are convinced that fosfomycin constituted a real benefit for patients with cystic fibrosis suffering from acute exacerbations of their chronic lung disease.

Zusammenfassung

Die Mukoviszidose ist die häufigste chronische Erbkrankheit bei Säuglingen und Kleinkindern und ist gekennzeichnet durch zähflüssiges Sekret aller exokrinen Drüsen. Die gestörte mukoziliäre Clearance führt über rezidivierende pulmonale Infekte zu irreversibler Lungenschädigung.

Gegenwärtig verfügbare Antibiotika zeigen oft geringe klinische Wirksamkeit aufgrund der hohen Resistenz der Keime insbesondere von Pseudomona aeruginosa und geänderter pharmakokinetischer Eigenheiten. Bei 86 (49 weiblichen und 37 männlichen) Patienten wurde Fosfomycin in einer klinischen Studie eingesetzt. Die antimikrobielle Empfindlichkeitsprüfung zeigte im Plättchentest ein hohes Maß an Resistenz gegen Fosfomycin. Im Diffusionstest wurde jedoch ein kleiner Teil der Stämme nachgetestet und ergab Werte, die deutlich im therapeutischen Bereich lagen. Dies und günstige therapeutische Ergebnisse in einer Pilotstudie ließen eine Fortsetzung der Studie zu.

Fosfomycin wurde als intravenöse Kurzinfusion von ca. 100 mg/kg Körpergewicht einmal täglich verabreicht. Die Verträglichkeit des Medikamentes war gut, es wurden keine Nebenwirkungen beobachtet. Die Beurteilung der Wirksamkeit von Fosfomycin bei pulmonalen Infekten bei Patienten mit Mukoviszidose ist schwierig. Eine Reihe von zusätzlichen Faktoren, wie Ernährung, Physikotherapie, beeinflussen das Befinden des Patienten zusätzlich zur antibiotischen Therapie. Außerdem wurde Fosfomycin vielfach in Kombination mit anderen Antibiotika verabreicht.

Besserung des Allgemeinbefindens, Gewichtszunahme, Verminderung des Sputums und Abnahme der Blutsenkungsgeschwindigkeit wurde jedoch bei ca. 65% der Patienten, die mit Fosfomycin als Monotherapie behandelt wurden, beobachtet. Der Prozentsatz klinischer Besserungen war bei Kombinationstherapie mit verschiedenen Antibiotika etwa gleich.

Auffallend war, daß insbesondere Patienten die deutliche Besserung durch die Gabe von Fosfomycin verspürten.

Die Diskrepanz der In-vitro-Resistenz mit guten klinischen Ergebnissen kann eventuell dadurch erklärt werden, daß eine Reihe von Pseudomonas-Stämmen in vivo empfindlich, in vitro jedoch resistent sind. Probleme der antimikrobiellen Empfindlichkeitsprüfung wurden beobachtet. Ein weiterer Faktor liegt eventuell darin, daß andere, fosfomycinempfindliche Keime klinische Relevanz besitzen.

Insgesamt scheint Fosfomycin bei akuten Exazerbationen von pulmonalen Infekten bei Patienten mit Mukoviszidose eine günstige klinische Wirksamkeit zu besitzen.

Introduction

Cystic fibrosis is the most frequent genetic syndrome of Caucasian infants and children. Cystic fibrosis has largely been a pediatric disease, but as time passes, increasing numbers of patients are surviving into adulthood. It is characterized by tenacious, viscid secretions of all exocrine glands, and an increased electrolyte content of sweat. The heterogeneity of this disorder is increasingly recognized in that it may be present as a primarily gastrointestinal, pulmonary, hepatic or reproductive disorder [2].

Pulmonary infection and obstruction result in most of the morbidity and over 90% of mortality. Almost all patients have some degree of chronic pulmonary obstruction and infection by Staphylococcus aureus and gramnegative organisms including various strains of pseudomonas. The early beginning of the disease is the mucopurulent bronchiolitis which often leads to obliterating bronchiolitis [3]. Due to the altered mucociliary clearance the major bronchi will then be involved by chronic bacterial colonization which can hardly be eliminated [4, 5]. The primary goal for therapy is reducing the injury and irreversible tissue destruction from chronic infection and minimizing and delaying the progression of the pulmonary damage as long as possible.

Various antibiotics have been used with little success in CF patients due to a high degree of resistance of bacterial organisms and alterations in pharmacokinetic properties [6]. Fosfomycin has been investigated in the treatment of pulmonary infections because of the broad antimicrobial spectrum of activity against frequent pathogens in CF patients and the expectation of a good tissue penetration.

Clinical Investigation

Material and Methods

In a series of 86 patients (49 females and 37 males) fosfomycin has been investigated in a clinical, therapeutical study.

The age of the patients is shown in Table 1:

Table 1

Age groups in years	n = **86**
0–5	1
5–10	13
10–15	27
15–20	28
20–25	13
25–37	4

2 patients were exluded from the study, having refused further treatment after the first fosfomycin infusion.

Bacteriologic results from sputum cultures are summarized in Table 2:

Table 2

Organism	Number of patients
Pseudomonas aeruginosa	27
Pseudomonas fluorescens	14
Pseudomonas aeruginosa and fluorescens	14
Pseudomonas aeruginosa and Staphyloc. aur.	10
Pseudomonas aeruginosa and H. influenzae	7
Pseudomonas, Staph. aur. and H. influenzae	2
Pseudomonas and various other organisms	3
Pseudomonas cepacia	1

A total of 78 patients harbored pseudomonas strains, 22 in various combinations with different other pathogenic organisms.

These findings are in close agreement with the literature where Pseudomonas aeruginosa is present in 90% of patients, staphylococci, H. influenzae, Klebsiella pneumoniae and Serratia marcescens in 10%.

The sensitivity of pseudomonas strains to fosfomycin in the examined samples of bronchial secretions was investigated by a disk diffusion test with 50 µg fosfomycin disks and addition of 50 µg G-6-P-D. There was an unexpected high resistance of Pseudomonas aeruginosa of 90%. This incidence of resistance may be partly induced by the high degree of mucoid strains in CF patients (70–80%) as compared to 0.9–2.0% in non-CF patients with pseudomonas infections. Other possibilities are problems of antimicrobial susceptibility testing with fosfomycin. In a later study 5 strains of pseudomonas insensitive to fosfomycin by disc diffusion were retested with an tube dilution test with Müller Hinton broth and all strains were well within the sensitive range.

Despite of this problems in antimicrobial susceptibility testing and the high degree of resistance of pseudomonas by disc diffusion methods, fosfomycin was found effective in early treatment trials and patients seemed to benefit greatly from this drug. The therapeutic investigation was therefore continued.

Fosfomycin was administered as infusion over 30–40 minutes once daily. The total dose varied from 15–262 g/patient, given in one to 5 courses between 1 and 4 years of treatment.

The dosage of fosfomycin was adjusted to body weight:

15–20 kg body weight	2.5 g/d
20–30 kg body weight	3.0 g/d
30–60 kg body weight	5.0 g/d
over 60 kg body weight	6.0 g/d

Duration of one course of fosfomycin treatment.

5–10 days	35 patients
10–15 days	42 patients
15–20 days	19 patients
20–25 days	13 patients
25–30 days	2 patients
30–35 days	3 patients

Duration depended on patients compliance, clinical results and local reactions of the veins.

The application of fosfomycin alone or in combination with a second antibiotic depended on treatment prior to admission, severity of the disease and the underlying bacterial flora:

Fosfomycin alone	20 patients
Fosfomycin + vibramycin	24 patients
Fosfomycin + aminoglycosides	5 patients
Fosfomycin + TMP Sulfa	23 patients
Fosfomycin + cephalosporin	
1st ° or penicillin	14 patients

Side effects from fosfomycin therapy were rare.

Dizziness	1
Eosinophilia	1
Phlebitis	5
Fever	2

In the two patients who developed fever during fosfomycin therapy it was explained by progressive deterioration due to the disease and not as drug fever.

Results

The results of fosfomycin therapy are difficult to evaluate objectively.

Change in environment, intensive supportive care and physiotherapy, adequate alimentation and additional drug therapy may already improve the condition of an individual patient by itself. The evaluation of the effect of fosfomycin in our series is therefore an arbitrary one, based on our experience in the treatment of many hundreds of CF patients.

Our parameters were: general condition, sputum and cough, body weight, blood sedimentation rate (ESR). The best indicator for the efficacy of a given antimicrobial agent in CF patients is the early improvement of the general condition and the rapid diminution of cough and bronchial secretion which is observed as early as 3–4 days after initiation of therapy.

Improvement of general condition,	
diminution of cough and sputum	79.76% of patients
No change under fosfomycin therapy	14.28% of patients
Deterioration of condition	5.95% of patients

Body weight was compared in 2 groups of patients; one treated with fosfomycin alone and one group with a combination of antibiotics:

	Combination therapy (%)	Monotherapy (%)
Increase in body weight	61.9	65
Decrease in body weight	20.2	20
Unchanged	17.8	15

Changes in body weight are highly dependent on the child's nutritional status and feeding problems during inpatient therapy. A change in ESR may indicate a certain degree of improvement of the lung function in CF patients. The incidence of such improvement corresponds prima vista to the increase in body weight. However, many of the patients with increase in body weight show normal ESRs, so that the different parameters are not congruent in a given patient benefitting from fosfomycin treatment. Results of changes in ESR are again divided into two groups.

	Combination therapy (%)	Monotherapy (%)
Decreased	64.93	65
Increased	19.48	20
Unchanged	15.58	15

In a few patients with recent deterioration and long-term fosfomycin treatment of at least 20 days improvement similar to that obtained with pseudomonas active cephalosporins or aminoglycosides has been observed.

10 patients of our series have died since the beginning of our clinical investigation 4 years ago.

Discussion

The prevalence of mucoid strains of pseudomonas is very high eventually inducing the mentioned degree of in vitro resistance to fosfomycin. Despite of these poor results in susceptibility testing a favorable clinical response has been obtained with fosfomycin in a substantial number of patients. It is particularly remarkable, that combination therapy did not offer any advantage over fosfomycin therapy alone. It is our firm believe but we cannot offer conclusive evidence yet that there are frequent strains of pseudomonas sensitive to fosfomycin in vivo. Another possibility to explain some of these favorable results is, that underlying bacteria other than pseudomonas with clinical relevance may be largely sensitive to fosfomycin. Problems in antimicrobial susceptibility testing have been described above.

Patients suffering from cystic fibrosis have the largest experience in antibiotic therapy. Nearly all of them who experienced improvement under fosfomycin indicated a rapid change in their condition with practically no side effects. We know that no antimicrobial agent will ever cure a CF patient and bacterial colonization is far from being inhibited.

But any drug which proves efficacious is highly welcome in the management of patients with cystic fibrosis.

Conclusion

We must admit, that in this pilot study, dosage and duration of fosfomycin therapy have not yet been adequate and should be reconsidered in great detail. Furthermore it has been difficult to assess the outcome of therapy as numerous different factors play a role.

Our choice of fosfomycin in the treatment of patients with cystic fibrosis may be summarized as follows:

A new class of antibiotics without cross resistance.

Simple parenteral administration even for outpatients.

Few side effects.

Favorable clinical response in the majority of patients even as monotherapy.

Large antibacterial spectrum. Despite of problems in antimicrobial susceptibility testing we feel, that there is a great potential in fosfomycin in the treatment of acute excerbations of pulmonary infections in patients with CF.

References

1. Matthews L, Drota D (1984) Cystic fibrous a long-term chronic disease. Ped Clin North Am 31: 133–152
2. Davis PB, di Sant'Agnese PA (1980) A review. Cystic fibrosis at fourty—Quo vadis? Pediatr Res 14: 83–87
3. Hoiby N (1982) Microbiology of lung infections in cystic fibrosis patients. Acta Paed Scand 301: 33–54
4. Doershuk CF, Stern RC (1985) Cystic fibrosis. In: Gellis SS, Kagan BM (eds) Current pediatric therapy. Saunders, Philadelphia
5. Hoiby N, Schiotz PO (1982) Immun complex mediated tissue damage in the lungs of cystic fibrosis with pseudomonas infection. Acta Paed Scand 301: 63–73
6. Guggenbichler JP, Pillwein K, Schabel F, Rohrer R (1981) Pharmakokinetik von Patienten mit Mukoviscidose. Pädiatr Pädol 16: 393–402

Author's address: Dr. H. Meyer, Alpine Kinderklinik Pro Juventute, CH-7272 Davos-Platz, Switzerland.

Fosfomycin in Pediatric Oncology

U. Bode, B. Hülsmann, M. Erps, und S. Soutadji

Universitäts-Kinderklinik, Bonn, Federal Republic of Germany

Summary

Children with leucemias or solid tumors receive intensive chemotherapy for periods of several months. Frequent infectious episodes require antimicrobial therapy for days or weeks. Surveillance cultures of pharynx, urine, vagina, rectum, and surface lesions as well as the antibiotic sensitivities were obtained three-weekly. In case of fever these specimen and multiple blood cultures were taken again. If physical examination and chest X-ray showed no signs of infection but neutropenia (500 granulocytes/mm^2 or less) the patients are started on broad spectrum antibiotic coverage. The regimen was changed if bacteriological results or clinical deterioration required it. Otherwise the patients was treated until neutropenia and fever subsided for at least two days.

Due to the emergence of oxacillin- and gentamicin resistant staphylococci in patients and medical care personnel fosfomycin was included in the antibiotic regimen. In over 100 febrile episodes fosfomycin (50 mg/kg body weight) was given in 8 hourly intervals in combination with cefotaxime, ceftazidime or ceftizoxime. In 25% of patients a bacterial infections was documented, while 75% of episodes had to be called fever of unknown origin (FUO) retrospectively. In the latter group two thirds of the patients were afebrile within 48 hours following antibiotic treatment. In one third of the patients fever subsided with the recovery of the bone marrow function. The combination of fosfomycin and a newer cephalosporine constitutes highly effective, nontoxic therapy for severe infections in immunocompromised patients.

Zusammenfassung

Die Behandlung der Leukämien und soliden Tumoren erfordert intensive Chemotherapie über mehrere Jahre. Die Erfahrung der letzten Jahre zeigte, daß die Intensität der antineoplastischen Chemotherapie direkt proportional mit der Erfolgsrate in der Tumorbekämpfung steht. Unter dieser intensiven Therapie muß jedoch notwendigerweise eine länger dauernde Knochenmarkdepression in Kauf genommen werden. Während man die Anämie bzw. die Thrombopenie durch gezielte Substitution behandeln kann, sind neutropenische Episoden und die daraus folgenden Infektionen zur führenden Nebenwirkung geworden. Autopsiebefunde zeigen, daß bei 80% der Todesfälle von Patienten mit Leukämie eine Infektion vorliegt. Infektionen sind teils tumor-, teils therapiebedingt. Die Keime, die isoliert werden, sind einerseits bakterielle Erreger: während in der letzten Dekade gramnegative Erreger und Pseudomonas überwogen, spielen in den letzten Jahren wiederum vermehrt grampositive Kokken, insbesonders koagulasepositive und koagulasenegative Staphylokokken, die zum Teil Oxacillin-/Gentamycinresistent sind, eine bedeutende Rolle. Daneben kommen auch Viren (CMV, Herpes), Pilze, Protozoen (Pneumocystis carinii, Toxoplasma) vor; Anaerobier sind im Gegensatz zu Erwachsenen im Hintergrund. Ein wesentlicher, prädisponierender Faktor für das Angehen einer Infektion ist eine Neutropenie. Bakterielle Erreger werden zwischen 15 und 25% febriler Episoden gezüchtet. Bei Patienten mit Leukozytenzahlen von weniger als 500 mm^3 gelingt dennoch nicht immer eine Keimisolation; man muß daher diese febrilen Episoden als Fieber ungeklärter Genese — eine wesentliche Komplikation in der pädiatrischen Onkologie — bezeichnen. Besonderer Wert muß auf persönliche Hygiene (Mundhygiene, Zahnsanierung, Stuhlhygiene) gelegt werden. Übersichtskulturen werden dreimal wöchentlich aus der Nase, der Mundhöhle, (bei älteren Kindern) Sputum, dem Harn, der Vagina, dem Rektum und eventuell von oberflächlichen Wunden abgenommen. Insbesondere die bakteriologische Überwachung der Stuhlflora mit Resistenzbestimmung der dominanten Keime, die in erster Linie die Quelle für eine endogene Infektion darstellen, ist wichtig. Beim Auftreten von Fieber werden mehrere Blutkulturen, ein Lungenröntgen und ein komplettes Blutbild durchgeführt. Eine antibiotische Behandlung mit Breitspektrum-Antibiotika ist jedoch bei Fieber immer nötig. Es war nun von Interesse, ob Fosfomycin — wegen des breiten Spektrums insbesondere gegen Staphylokokken — in Kombination mit einem Cephalosporin in der Behandlung von febrilen Episoden bei immunsupprimierten, neutropenischen Patienten eine Bereicherung der Behandlungsmöglichkeiten darstellt.

100 fieberhafte Episoden mit Keimnachweis oder Fieber unklarer Genese wurde mit Fosfomycin (50 mg/kg Körpergewicht) alle 8 Stunden behandelt. Es erfolgte eine Kombination mit einem Cephalosporin der 3 Generation Cefotaxim, Ceftazidim oder Ceftizoxim. Bei 25% der Fälle wurde eine bakterielle Infektion dokumentiert. Bei 21 von 25 Infektionen wurde ein therapeutischer Erfolg verzeichnet. 75% waren Fieberschübe

unklarer Genese. In der zweiten Gruppe waren zwei Drittel der Patienten innerhalb von 48 Stunden fieberfrei. Bei einem Drittel der Patienten kam es im Rahmen der Knochenmarkregeneration zum Fieberabfall. Die Kombination von Fosfomycin mit einem Cephalosporin der 3. Generation ist bei immunsupprimierten Patienten mit schweren bakteriellen Infektionen eine wirksame Therapie ohne substantielle Nebenwirkungen.

Introduction

In contrast to the therapeutic concepts in adult oncology the basic approach in pediatric oncology is the maximal delivery of cytotoxic agents over a short time span, while surgery and radiotherapy are mostly adjuvant therapeutic modalities. The experience of the last 10–15 years showed that the intensity of treatment correlated closely with the therapeutic success rate. Thus, drug concentrations are chosen which empirically result in a tolerable level of toxicity and warrant the overall success rate of 66% in children treated for cancer.

With the intensity of cytotoxic treatment obligatorily bone marrow depression is observed. The effects of anemia and thrombocytopenia may be compensated by substitution of blood products. The leucopenia, however, results in frequent infections, the major side effects of chemotherapy today. Autopsy results indicate that 80% of the leukemic patients and 50% of the patients with solid tumors show signs of infections at the time of death. Half of the patients have a documented sepsis and 50% show pneumonia in addition. Analysing the microbiological source, a bacterial origin is documented in ⅔ of the bacteremic patients and in 40% of the patients with pneumonia.

Infections in Immunosuppressed Patients

The intensity of the treatment and the damage by the disease itself predisposes the oncological patient to infections (Table 1). Disease-related are the effects of the tumor on the function of lymphocytes as it is in lymphoma and Hodgkin disease in particular. Infiltration of the bone marrow by the disease leads to a quantitative deficiency of

Table 1. Infections: Predispositions of oncological patients

A. Disease-related

---

1. Immune system
   a) qualitative (Hodgkin, NHL)
   b) quantitative (BM infiltration)
2. Infiltration (skin, mucosa)
3. Obstruction (respir., GI, UG tract)
4. Weight loss

Table 2. Infections: Predispositions of oncological patients

B. Therapy-related

---

1. Surface lesions (surgery, irradiation, chemotherapy)
2. BM depression (chemotherapy, rarely irradiation)
   a) qualitative (phagocytosis, migration, lymphocytes)
   b) quantitative
3. Supportive care
   a) antibiotics
   b) blood products
   c) nosocomial infections

---

the bone marrow reserve. Tumor infiltration of skin and mucosa may be another port of entry for infections.

Obstruction of excretory ways in the respiratory, urogenital or gastrointestinal tract by the tumor is another source of infection. Last but not least the poor nutritional status of patients with cancer predisposes them to infectious episodes.

More important, however, is the therapy-related infectious predisposition (Table 2). Surgical wounds, ulcerations of skin and mucosa caused by radiotherapy or chemotherapy lead to an increased risk of infections. Immunological studies have shown that phagocytosis and migration of granulocytes is impaired after chemotherapy. The most obvious effect is the quantitative reduction of the bone marrow capacity which leads to profound

Table 3. Infections

Bacterial	gram + and gram— bacteria; anerobic bacteria rare in pediatrics
Viral	Herpes simplex Varicella-zoster CMV, EBV measles
Fungal	candida cryptococci aspergillus phycomycoses
Protozoal	toxoplasma Pneumocystis carinii

neutropenia. Often forgotten are the dangers inherent in many measures of supportive care: frequent administration of antibiotics result in fungal growth and microbiological resistance, administration of blood products contains the risk of hepatitis and CMV infections, frequent hospitalization of patients exposes them to nosocomial infections characterized by resistance to most antibiotics.

Table 3 is a summary of the most important organisms causing infections in immunosuppressed patients. Bacterial infections are predominant. Back in 1960–1970, the grampositive bacteria dominated the list, while in the last decade gramnegative bacteria became more prominent. In recent years, however, staphylococci are reported to be an increasing problem. In contrast to adult oncology anerobic bacteria rarely occur in pediatric oncology. In any infectious episode it must be considered that fever may also be caused by viral, fungal or protozoal organisms. Herpes simplex and Zoster infections are less threatening sice the introduction of acyclovir therapy and the availability of a hyperimmunglobulin for CMV infections. For pediatricians measles infections in oncology patients are still a nightmare, but the thorough information of

parents and the early and generous prophylaxis with commercial
IgG products which contain considerable measle titers make it a
rare event. Fungal infections are fortunately also rare as they occur
mostly in patients after bone marrow transplantations or other

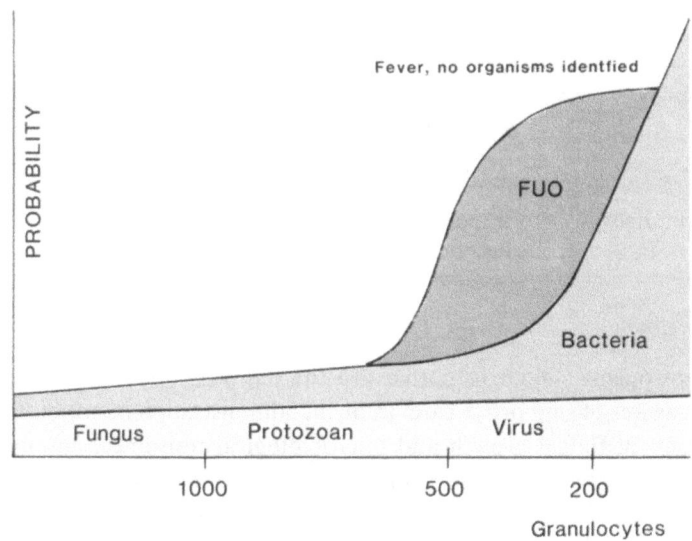

Fig. 1. Probability of infectious agents dependent on granulocyte counts in
children with cancer

prolonged aplasias. The introduction of cotrimoxazol prophylaxis
has reduced the risk of pneumocystis carinii pneumonia in leukemia
patients considerably.

Fig. 1 shows a scheme of the relationship between granulocyte
count and probability of infectious organisms. The occurrence of
viral, fungal, and protozoal diseases is dependent on general
immunsuppression and does not correlate strongly with the absolute neutrophil count (ANC). There is always a risk of bacterial
infections and it increases dramatically below an ANC of 500.
Patient with neutrophil counts in the range of a few hundred, often
have fever but no organisms can be isolated or identified as the cause

of infections. This fever of unknown origin (FUO) is a major complication in pediatric oncology. Former studies have shown that broad-spectrum antibiotic coverage is necessary for these patients until fever and neutropenia have subsided. In our hospital semisynthetic penicillins and aminoglycosides were used for antibiotic coverage for years. About two years ago the emergence of oxacillin- and gentamycin-resistant staphylococci required a change in the antibiotics regimen. The results of one hundred episodes of infection in children with cancer treated with a combination of fosfomycin and a cephalosporine of the third generation are presented.

Clinical Investigation

Patients

One hundred febrile episodes occurred in 31 males and 15 females, 7 months to 21 years of age. The underlying diseases were malignancies of the hematopoetic system and solid tumors which were all treated with intensive chemotherapy. Acute lymphoblastic leukemia is the most common malignant disease in childhood and therefore prominent in the patient collective (Table 4).

Table 4. Diagnosis

Leukemias	27	Solid tumors	19
ALL	13	osteosarcoma	6
AML	3	Ewing sarcoma	2
CML	2	rhabdomyosarcoma	2
NHL	8	brain tumors	4
Histiocytosis X	1	testicular carcinoma	1
		chondrosarcoma	1
		hepatoblastoma	1
		Wilms tumor	1
		hemangiopericytoma	1

Table 5. Prophylaxis

Personal hygiene
Dental status
Care of lesions
Surveillance cultures (3-weekly)
Antibiotics
Viral serology
Immunoglobulines

Prophylactic Measures

To prevent infectious episodes in our patients, we stress prophylactic regimens, in which patients and nursing staff are involved (Table 5). Patients are informed about the importance of personal hygiene. At the beginning of oncological treatment the dental status is evaluated and, if necessary, corrected. Skin and mucosal lesions are carefully treated. One example is the prevention of constipation by laxatives in order to prevent lesions of the anal ring by hard stool consistency. Routinely, microbiological cultures are taken of the nose and throat, sputum (in older children), urine, stool and skin lesions. As it is known that most infections are caused by endogenous organisms, this routine supplies information on probable infectious causes and their antibiotic sensitivity. Patients with hematological malignancies receive cotrimoxazol as prophylaxis against pneumocystis carvinic infections during the intensive period of their tratment. During these episodes polymyxin-E is given for intestinal decontamination and nystatine to prevent fungal colonization. In patients with solid tumors and documented colonization oral nystatine is given, too. If no plasma products are given, titers against the above mentioned viral strains are determined every three months. We object to the routine administration of immunoglobulines, reserving it for limited indications.

Diagnostic Measures

A patient with fever is thoroughly examined whereby neutropenia may change the picture of clinical presentation. For instance, a

Table 6. Antibiotics

Fosfomycin IV Q 8 hours (120–250 mg/kg/day)	
+ Ceftizoxime IV Q 8 hours (100–150 mg/kg/day)	5
+ Cefotaxime IV Q 8 hours (100–150 mg/kg/day)	43
+ Ceftazidime IV Q 8 hours (100–150 mg/kg/day)	52
Total	100 episodes

perirectal infection will lack swelling and abscess formation only showing the symptoms of itching and mild local erythema. A chest X-ray is performed if there is the slightest indication for a respiratory tract infection. Cultures and serology are taken again and several blood cultures are obtained. Blood cultures are repeated if fever recurs or if the clinical status deteriorates. The CBS is determined with special attention to the neutrophil count. If the ANC is below 500, intravenous antibiotic treatment is given regardless of the clinical status of the patient. Nonneutropenic patients are treated with antibiotics only if they are clinically ill.

Antibiotic Treatment

In one hundred febrile episodes fosfomycin was given in combination with a cephalosporine of the third generation (Table 6). The antibiotics were given intravenously every eight hours. For fosfomycin the single dose was 50 mg/kg with a maximum dose of 3 g. The cephalosporine dose was 50 mg/kg with a maximum dose of 2 g. This antibiotic regimen was only chosen for those patients in whom the surveillance cultures and the antibiotic sensitivities did no require a different preferential regimen. For instance, if enterococci were found in stool cultures, these patients were not included, as this regimen is known to be less effective against these organisms.

Leucocyte Counts

The obligatory antibiotic therapy of children with cancer depends on the absolute neutrophil count (ANC). Table 7 shows the

Table 7. CBS Neutropenia (granulocytes < 500) 87 patients

Leucocytes:		
	< 500	38 patients
	500–1,000	22 patients
	1,000–2,000	20 patients
	> 2,000	7 patients

No neutropenia 13 patients (4 documented infections).

Table 8. Results

Antibiotic success		
Documented infections		21
Nonneutropenic	4	
Neutropenic	17	
Afebrile within 48 hours		19
DOD, febrile, negative BC		2

leucocyte counts in all patients. It is known that even young children show neutrophil dominance while receiving chemotherapy so that the number of neutrophils constantly decreases following chemotherapy and slowly increases after passing the nadir of bone marrow depression. The reticulocyte count is a sensitive parameter of bone marrow activity, correlating well with low ANCs. Several patients with higher leucocyte counts demonstrate high peripheral blast counts. When fever as the only reliable sign of infection occurred, the majority of patients exhibited severe bone marrow depression.

Documented Infections

In 21 of 100 febrile episodes blood or CSF cultures were positive (Table 8). 19 of the 21 patients were afebrile within 46 hours, 2 children continued to have fever in spite of negative blood cultures and died of their disease.

13 fever episodes in nonneutropenic patients were treated with antibiotics and fever subsided within 48 hours in all of them. Four of

Table 9. Results

Fever in patients > 500 ANC		13
Documented infections		4
Blood: gramnegative rods	1	
Staphylococcus epidermidis	3	
CSF: Staphylococcus epidermidis	1	
Afebrile within 48 hours		13

Table 10. Results

Neutropenic < 500 ANC		87
Documented infections		17
Blood: Staphylococcus aureus	8	
Staphylococcus epidermidis	1	
streptococci	4	
CSF: Staphylococcus aureus	1	
Staphylococcus epidermidis	3	
Fever of unknown origin (FUO)		70

these 13 patients suffered from sepsis, caused by gramnegative rods in one instance and coagulasenegative staphylococci in 3 cases. One of these also had a CSF infection (Table 9).

In 17 of 87 febrile episodes in patients with ANCs less than 500 positive blood or CSF cultures were obtained (Table 10).

Sepsis was caused by Staphylococcus aureus (8 patients), by Staphylococcus epidermidis (1 patient), and streptococci (4 patients). In CSF coagulasenegative staphylococci were documented in three instances and one CSF sample showed Staphylococcus aureus. It should be mentioned that several patients had a ventricular-atrial shunt for hydrocephalus explaining the frequent occurrence of Staphylococcus epidermidis in CSF.

Neutropenia and FUO

In 70 episodes neutropenia and fever of unknown origin (FUO) was documented. Though no organism could be identified in these cases,

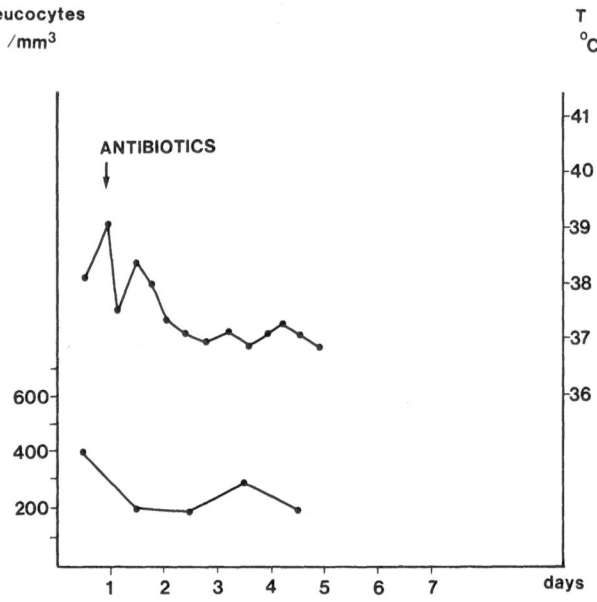

Fig. 2. Fever and neutropenia, antibiotic effect

empirical data have documented the necessity of broad-spectrum antibiotic coverage. Even if fever persists this treatment prevents superinfections during the phase of neutropenia. Antibiotic therapy should be stopped when fever subsides for longer than 48 hours and/or neutropenia is no longer present.

Thus three types of responses to antibiotic treatment can be differentiated. Antibiotics were considered effective if fever subsided within 48 hours in spite of continued neutropenia (Fig. 2). If fever persisted in spite of antibiotics as long as neutropenia was present, recovery was not considered due to antibiotics but to bone marrow recovery (Fig. 3). It has to be mentioned, however, that the antibiotics most likely prevented superinfections and therefore cannot be considered ineffective. In several patients neutropenia and fever continued for several days in spite of treatment (Fig. 4). It

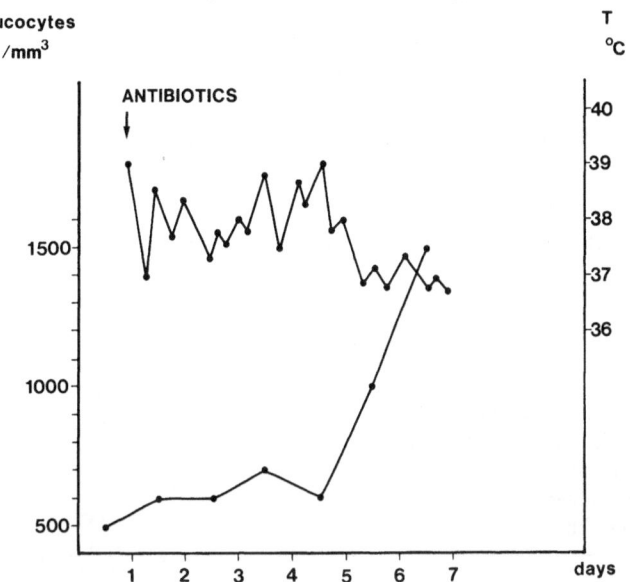

Fig. 3. Fever and neutropenia, no antibiotic effect, BM recovery

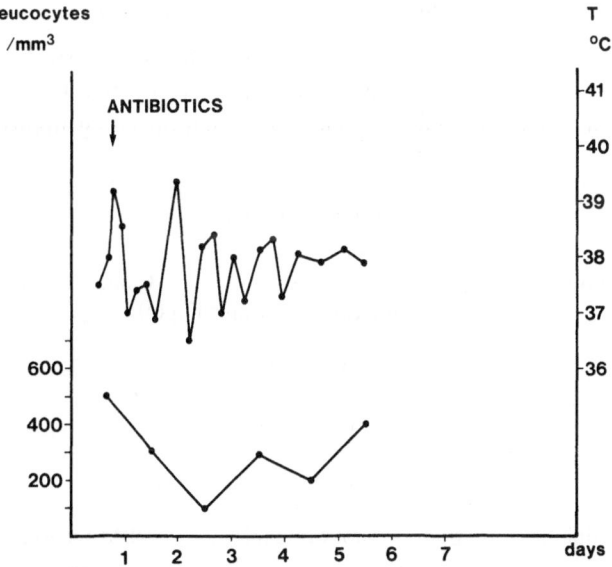

Fig. 4. Fever and neutropenia, antibiotic effect not evaluable

is obvious that neither antibiotics nor bone marrow recovery contributed to defervescence. These cases are labeled "not evaluable antibiotic effect".

41 of 70 patients with FUO were afebrile within 48 hours after the start of antibiotic therapy. In 21 instances bone marrow recovery was considered responsible for defervescence. 7 episodes were not evaluable for antibiotic effect. One patient died of disease (Table 11).

Table 11. Results

FUO in neutropenia	70
Afebrile within < 48 hours	41
BM recovery	21
Not evaluable	7
DOD, febrile	1

Prior Ineffective Antibiotic Treatment

7 patients had received other antibiotics before the start of this regime and continued to have fever and neutropenia. Cefuroxime (2) and ampicillin (5) were given in combination with gentamycin. 5

Table 12. Results

Persistant fever	→	Change of antibiotics
cefuroxime (2)	ampicillin (5)	
	+	
	gentamycin (7)	
	↓	
	fosfomycin	
	+	
	3rd generation cephalosporin	
antibiotic response (5)	not evaluable (1)	BM recovery (1)

Table 13. Side effects of fosfomycin

Resistance development	
Microbiological:	Staphylococcus epidermidis 1
Toxicity	
Allergic reactions:	not observed
Organ toxicity:	not observed

patients were afebrile within 48 hours after fosfomycin and cephalosporin therapy, while bone marrow recovery and no evaluable effect of antibiotics were each documented in one patient (Table 12).

During the antibiotic treatment a strain of Staphylococcus epidermidis developed resistance to fosfomycin. Fortunately, this was clinically irrelevant, since the strain was sensitive to the combination partner of fosfomycin.

In all epidodes laboratory parameters of liver and kidney function were controlled besides the bone marrow activity. Though organ dysfunction was present before commencement of antibiotic treatment, no toxicity of this regimen on any organ was observed. There were no signs of allergic reactions so that the combination of fosfomycin and a cephalosporin seems to be nontoxic (Table 13).

Summary

In summary 100 febrile episodes in young cancer patients were treated with a combination of fosfomycin and a new cephalosporin. Though nearly all of the patients were neutropenic (< 500), 69% were afebrile within 48 hours after initiation of antibiotic therapy. 21% showed defervescence after bone marrow recovery, three patients died of their disease with continuing fever but without documented infection. In seven episodes an obvious antibiotic effect could not be recognized. The microbiologically identified organisms of septic diseases were mostly grampositive organisms which were eliminated totally by this antibiotic regimen. The low occurrence of toxicity and resistance development is another positive aspect of this combination chemotherapy.

Authors' address: Dr. U. Bode, Universitäts-Kinderklinik und Poliklinik Bonn, Adenauerallee, D-5300 Bonn 1, Federal Republic of Germany.

Fosfomycin in the Treatment of Infections Difficult to Treat

W. Marget and K. Lohse

Infectious Disease Division, University Childrens Hospital, München,
Federal Republic of Germany

Summary

At the University of Munich Childrens Hospital 40 children with severe infections were treated with fosfomycin in 1980. The age range of the patients was 4 weeks to 16 years (average age 7.5 years).

9 patients with septicemia, 11 with shunt infections and ventriculitis, 3 with pneumonia, 8 with osteomyelitis, 6 with cystic fibrosis and 3 with various other diseases were enrolled in this therapeutic investigation. Virtually all patients have received previous unsuccessful antimicrobial therapy with cephalosporines 3rd generation and/or aminoglycosides before fosfomycin was considered. The treatment was well tolerated in every instance, no side effects were observed.

In the treatment of patients with septicemia, it is necessary to administer an adequate dose of fosfomycin, i.e., 200 mg/kg body weight. Of 11 patients with shunt infections and ventriculitis all patients showed a clinical and bacteriological response; also 7 of 8 patients with osteomyelitis were successfully treated. 5 of 6 patients with cystic fibrosis were successfully treated. Less satisfactory results were achieved in immunocompromized patients with nosocomial infections: only 4 of 9 patients responded to fosfomycin therapy in combination with aminoglycosides or 3rd generation cephalosporines. The highest rate of cure was observed in infections due to Staphylococcus aureus and Staphylococcus epidermidis with 15 of 18 patients. These data show, that we have not yet fully exhausted the possibilities of fosfomycin therapy in view of its efficacy and good tolerance.

Zusammenfassung

An der Universitäts-Kinderklinik München wurde bei 40 Patienten mit verschiedenen, schwer zu behandelnden Infekten Fosfomycin eingesetzt. Alle Patienten waren bereits mit verschiedenen Antibiotika, meist der Kombination eines Aminoglykosids, mit einem Cephalosporin der 3. Generation erfolglos vorbehandelt. Bei diesen Patienten handelte es sich um Säuglinge, Kleinkinder und ältere Kinder im Alter zwischen 4 Monaten und 16 Jahren.

Bei 9 Patienten bestand eine Sepsis, bei 11 eine Infektion eines Spitz-Holter-Ventils mit Ventrikulitis, bei 8 Patienten wurde eine akute hämatogene Osteomyelitis diagnostiziert, bei 3 Patienten eine Pneumonie und bei 9 verschiedene andere Infekte; 6 dieser Kinder hatten eine Mukoviszidose. Das Ziel dieser Untersuchung war es, festzustellen, ob
1. eine klinische bzw. bakteriologische Heilung erzielt werden kann,
2. eine rationelle Gesamt-Tagesdosis angegeben werden kann, und
3. die Verträglichkeit des Präparates gegeben ist.

Fosfomycin wurde bei allen Patienten in einer Gesamt-Tagesdosis von 200–250 mg/kg Körpergewicht intravenös verabreicht. Frühere Therapieversuche mit einer Gesamttagesdosis von 100 mg/kg Körpergewicht waren wegen der zu niedrigen Dosis nicht aussagekräftig. Eine Steigerung der Tagesdosis ist wegen der großen therapeutischen Breite des Medikamentes unproblematisch. Fosfomycin wurde auch bei den Patienten in dieser Untersuchung ausgezeichnet vertragen. Es wurden keine Nebenwirkungen beobachtet.

Die Behandlungsergebnisse zeigten bei allen 11 behandelten Patienten mit Shunt-Infektion einen ausgezeichneten Erfolg. Auch 7 von 8 Patienten mit Osteomyelitis konnten erfolgreich behandelt werden, wie auch 2 von 3 Patienten mit Pneumonie. Von 6 Patienten mit einer akuten pulmonalen Exazerbationen bei Mukoviszidose und Pseudomonas aeruginosa als dominantem Keim wurde bei 5 Patienten eine klinische Besserung, Abnahme des Sputums, Entfieberung beobachtet. Relativ schlecht waren die Behandlungsergebnisse bei immunsupprimierten Patienten mit nosokomialen gramnegativen Infekten: nur 4 von 9 Patienten konnten erfolgreich behandelt werden, wobei jedoch anzumerken ist, daß all diese Patienten bereits antibiotisch mit hochwirksamen Antibiotika vorbehandelt waren. Insgesamt konnten 30 von 40 infektiösen Episoden klinisch erfolgreich behandelt werden.

Die bakteriologischen Ergebnisse waren bei Staphylokokken, und zwar sowohl bei koagulasepositiven Keimen (10 von 12) als auch bei koagulasenegativen Stämmen (5 von 6) gut. Geringer war die Wirksamkeit gegen gramnegative Erreger, wobei hier nur 7 von 13 Keimen erfolgreich eliminiert werden konnte.

Zusammenfassend kann festgestellt werden, daß Fosfomycin bei schweren, bakteriellen, nosokomialen Infekten bei verschiedenen Grundkrankheiten (Fremdkörperinfektion mit Ventrikulitis, Mukoviszidose) als Alternativmedikament Beachtung verdient. Die gute Gewebspenetration und Verträglichkeit sowie die Möglichkeit der Kombination mit Aminoglykosiden oder neuen Cephalosporinen eröffnet theapeutische Möglichkeiten bei schwer zu behandelnden bzw. erfolglosen Fällen.

Introduction

The antimicrobial activity of fosfomycin covers a large spectrum of pathogenic and opportunistically pathogenic organisms. Since no parallel resistance is to be expected, this drug occupies a unique position among available chemotherapeutics. The well-known advantages of this substance, namely its low toxicity and good tissue penetration particularly into the meninges and bone in comparison with other antibiotics makes it especially valuable for use in children. The wide safe dosage range is advantageous in regard to the various age groups and the frequent occurrence of dehydration. For the pediatrician the main shortcoming of this substance is its high sodium content which makes monitoring of electrolytes mandatory when administered in high doses to neonates and infants. For this reason we consider the aversion to this medication that has prevailed in central Europe and the USA for many years as unjustified. However, discrepancies exist between the results of microbiological tests and clinical success. It should also be emphasized, that little can be learned from the results of oral administration obtained many years ago. Retrospectively the original dosage of 100–200 mg/kg body weight/day for children and infants proved to be too low; our recommended dosage now is 200–250 mg/kg body weight/day.

A major field of application is in nosocomial infections, particularly due to coagulase negative staphylococci and Staphylococcus aureus where other antibiotics may have failed.

The considerations were underscored by more recent findings, most notable by Kazmierzak and Portier who recommend a combination of fosfomycin with cefotaxim as an effective regimen

Table 1. Fosfomycin susceptibility (%)

	Staph. aureus		Staph. epidermis		E. coli	
	n	% s.	n	% s.	n	% s.
1978	94	97	128	73	238	49
1979	165	95	194	83	331	98
1980	233	97	255	75	501	98
1981	229	97	281	84	456	98
1982	249	98	161	78	393	99
1983	174	96	80	74	351	100
1984	304	94	104	68	385	99

in the treatment of Spitz-Holter's valve infection. A Danish group headed by Nissen regards the combination of fosfomycin and ampicillin in critically ill patients as superior to presently recommended treatment regimen. Since this antibiotic was first placed at our disposal, no change in resistance situation of the most important agents of nosocomial infections at our clinic have been observed in routine agar diffusion tests. The same applies to the MIC determinations (Table 1).

Clinical Investigaion

We present a casuistic retrospective study of 40 cases of severe, difficult to treat or refractory infections. The objective of this approach was to decide whether the inclusion of fosfomycin in the routine therapeutic regimen in our clinic is advisable.

Patient Profile

40 treatments were carried out in 29 children, the majority of whom showed compromised host responses. Their age range of our patients was 4 weeks to 16 years, with a mean age of 7.5 years. Treatment was commenced at the end of 1980.

Included were 9 patients with sepsis, 11 patients with infected

Spitz-Holter valve, 3 patients with pneumonia, 8 patients with osteomyelitis, and 9 patients with various other diseases among them 6 patients with cystic fibrosis and serious pulmonary exacerbation of their chronic lung infection. Pseudomonas aeruginosa was the dominant organism in these patients. Antimicrobial susceptibility of the causative pathogens was first determined by an agar diffusion method and in addition MIC testing was performed. In the majority of cases fosfomycin therapy had been preceded by conventional therapy with aminoglycosides and 3rd generation cephalosporins without success.

The efficacy of therapy was documented by means of clinical parameters such as body temperature, ESR, leucocyte count, differential blood count and bacteriological investigations.

The following points were taken into account:

1. Was fosfomycin dosage sufficient and was eradication of the causative organism achieved with fosfomycin?

2. Was clinical cure achieved by fosfomycin?

3. Were side effects observed?

Results

Clinical Evaluation

Fosfomycin was well tolerated in every instance. No side effects were observed; particularly no electrolyte disturbance was observed. In Spitz-Holter shunt infection the therapy was considered successful if the patients were free of symptoms after 8 days of treatment. All children treated with fosfomycin showed a favorable outcome (Table 2). Fosfomycin therapy was successful in 7 of 8 patients with osteomyelitis (Table 3).

Two of three patients with pneumonia were also successfully treated (Table 4). In 5 of 6 patients with cystic fibrosis improvement was found in terms of fever, sputum quantity and quality and the results of blood tests (Table 5).

The poorest results were found in nosocomial sepsis with only 4 successful treated patients of 9 (Table 6). It has to be emphasized

Table 2. Clinical results—Spitz-Holter-drainage infection

Total n			Success			Side effects
			Clin. + bact.	Only clin.	Only bact.	
11	Staph. aureus	5	7	2	2	none
	Staph. epid.	5				
	Strept. d.	1				

Table 3. Clinical results—osteomyelitis

Total n			Clinical success	Side effects
8	Staph. aureus	2	7 not judgeable 1	none
	H. influencae	1		
	Proprioni bact.	1		
	Serratia	1		
	No isolation	3		

Table 4. Clinical results—pneumonia

Total number	3
Clinical success	2
Failure	1
Side effects	none

Table 5. Clinical results—other diseases (6 cystic fibrosis)

Total n			Success clin. + bact.	Side effects
9	Staph. aureus	1	6	none
	Pseudomonas	6		
	No isolation	2		

Table 6. Clinical results—sepsis

Total n			Success			Side-effects
			Clinical	Bact.	Clin. + bact.	
9	Serratia	1				
	Staph. aureus	5				
	H. influencae	1	4	4	4	none
	Pseudomonas	1				
	Staph. epid.	1				

again that all these patients have been pretreated with cephalosporines 3rd generation and aminoglycosides.

Our results show that infections due to Staphylococcus aureus and Staphylococcus epidermidis has the highest rate of cure with 10 of 12 and 5 of 6 strains respectively. Despite demonstrated susceptibility the cure rate for gramnegative organisms was substantially poorer, i.e., 7 of 13 cases. An overall clinical success was seen in 30 patients.

Conclusion

The results achieved in severe nosocomial infections show that fosfomycin represents an equivalent alternative to present therapeutic regimen in many cases. It is our firm believe that a prospective, comparative, randomized study in the treatment of severe nosocomial infections in children should be conducted in which established therapeutic regimen such as ampicillin in combination with aminoglycosides or vancomycin + rifampin, or an aminoglycoside combined with a cephalosporin 3rd generation are compared to fosfomycin in various combinations (e.g., aminoglycosides or cephalosporines 3rd generation). The strength of this substance appears to lie particularly in the treatment of infections with coagulasepositive und coagulasenegative staphylococci.

In view of the good tolerance of fosfomycin and its low toxicity, the broad antimicrobial activity and the absence of cross-resistance as our therapeutic results also demonstrate, fosfomycin is still unjustifyably neglected.

References

1. Kazmierzak A, Pechinot A, Tremeaux C, Muez JM, Kohli E, Portier H (1985) Bacterizidal activity of cefotaxime and fosfomycin in cerebro-spinal fluid during treatment of rabbit meningitis experimentally induced by methicillin resistant Staphylococcus aureus. Infection 13: 76–80
2. Portier H, Tremeaux JC, Chavanet P, Gouyon JB, Duez JM, Kazmier-zak A (1984) Treatment of severe staphylococcal infections with cefotaxime and fosfomycin in combination. J Antimicrob Chemoth 14 [Suppl] B: 277–284
3. Nissen LR, Jacobsen J, Raven T, Vahlgreen C, Auning-Hausen H (1986) Fosfomycin-Ampicillin versus Gentamicin-Ampiallin in the treatment of Critically ill pattients with pneumonia. Infection 14: 246–249

Authors' address: Dr. W. Marget, Infectious Disease Division, University Childrens Hospital, Lindwurmstrasse 4, D-8000 München, Federal Republic of Germany.

List of Contributors

Prof. Dr. *R. Achatzy*, Thorax- und Gefäßchirurgie, Speziallungenklinik Hemer, Postfach 360/380, D-5870 Hemer, Federal Republic of Germany.

Prof.-Doz. Dr. *U. Bode*, Universitätskinderklinik und Poliklinik, Adenauerallee 119, D-5300 Bonn 1, Federal Republic of Germany.

Doz. Dr. *J.-P. Guggenbichler*, Universitätsklinik für Kinderheilkunde, Anichstrasse 35, A-6020 Innsbruck, Austria.

Dr. *P. Höger*, Universität Hamburg, Kinderklinik, Neugeborenenstation, Martinistrasse 52, D-2000 Hamburg 20, Federal Republic of Germany.

Prof. Dr. *F. H. Kayser*, Institut für Medizinische Mikrobiologie, Universität Zürich, Gloriastrasse 32, CH-8028 Zürich, Switzerland.

Prof. Dr. *Ch. Krüger*, II. Med. Klinik Abt. 81, Medizinische Hochschule Lübeck, Ratzeburger Allee 160, D-2400 Lübeck, Federal Republic of Germany.

Prof. Dr. *W. Marget*, Kinderklinik im Dr. von Haunerschen Kinderhospital, Lindwurmstrasse 4, D-8000 München 2, Federal Republic of Germany.

Dr. *H. Meyer*, Höhenklinik Sanitas, CH-7270 Davos-Platz, Switzerland.

Prof. Dr. *H. J. Peters*, Urologische Abteilung, St.-Elisabeth-Krankenhaus, D-5000 Köln-Hohenlind, Federal Republic of Germany.

Priv.-Doz. Dr. *G. Pfeiffer*, Institut für Anästhesiologie, Universität Bonn, Sigmund-Freud-Strasse 25, D-5300 Bonn 1, Federal Republic of Germany.

Priv.-Doz. Dr. *B. Roth*, Bezirksspital Wattenwil, CH-3135 Wattenwil, Switzerland.

Dr. *H. Tritthart*, Universitätsklinik für Neurochirurgie, Auenbruggerplatz, A-8036, Austria.